Domestic Violence Treatment for Abusive Women

Domestic Violence Treatment for Abusive Women

A Treatment Manual

Ellen L. Bowen, LCSW, BCD

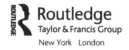

Routledge
Taylor & Francis Group
New York London

Routledge
Taylor & Francis Group
711 Third Avenue
New York, NY 10017

Routledge
Taylor & Francis Group
2 Park Square
Milton Park, Abingdon
Oxon OX14 4RN

© 2009 by Taylor & Francis Group, LLC
Routledge is an imprint of Taylor & Francis Group, an Informa business

International Standard Book Number-13: 978-0-7890-3811-1 (Softcover) 978-0-7890-3810-4 (Hardcover)

Library of Congress Cataloging-in-Publication Data

Bowen, Ellen L.
   Domestic violence treatment for abusive women : a treatment manual / by Ellen L. Bowen.
      p. ; cm.
   Includes bibliographical references and index.
   ISBN 978-0-7890-3810-4 (hardback : alk. paper) -- ISBN
   978-0-7890-3811-1 (pbk. : alk. paper)
   1. Abusive women--Rehabilitation. 2. Group psychotherapy. I. Title.
   [DNLM: 1. Domestic Violence--prevention & control. 2. Psychotherapy,
Group--methods. 3. Spouse Abuse--therapy. 4. Women--psychology. HV 6626 B7856d
2008]

RC569.5.F3B69 2008
616.85'822--dc22
                                               2008030167

Visit the Taylor & Francis Web site at
http://www.taylorandfrancis.com

and the Routledge Web site at
http://www.routledge.com

For my family, my teachers:

My parents, Ruth and Vernon, who continue to teach me the significance of attachment and the meaning of family. I am loved.

My siblings, Elise, Matt, and Heidi, who remind me that enjoying life doesn't depend on where you are, what you have, or what you are doing, but whom you are with. I am accepted.

My husband, Chris, the most consistent and patient person I have ever known. I am safe, secure.

My children, Meredith and Andrew, who stretch me, humble me, and give me perspective. I am proud.

My colleague, mentor, role model, adopted sister, second mom, and longtime treasured friend, Susan Schramm. I am privileged.

My clients over many years, who have shown courage in their willingness to be vulnerable and share with me their most private secrets. I am honored.

I am who I am because of your influence on me. I am blessed, and I am grateful.

Contents

PART 2 Practice

Introduction

I never expected to be doing therapy with abusive women.

As a clinical social worker, I had extensive experience with wives, girl-friends, and children of violent men. I thought domestic violence was a sociocultural problem characterized by men's use of power and control to batter their female partners: men were the perpetrators; women were the powerless victims.

Then, in 1997, two colleagues and I co-founded NOVA, Non-Violent Alternatives, a 52-week treatment program for domestic violence offenders. Months into my first group for abusive men, I was challenged to rethink my previously held beliefs about domestic violence.

A very proper elderly gentleman let slip more details about the argument that led to his arrest: before he had pushed his wife down, she had first head-butted him and then bit his nipple, drawing blood. He never told the police, his probation officer, or me because he was embarrassed. He thought that being a gentleman meant protecting his wife from the humiliation of jail, court, and so forth. To admit that he had been assaulted many times before by his wife would be like admitting that he was weak and unmanly. He was appalled by his own ungentlemanly behavior and ashamed because he had been raised to never hit a woman.

I was hearing more stories of women's threats, intimidation, and violence—too many to dismiss as simply "victim blaming." In many cases, the men's accounts of the violence in their relationships were corroborated by their wives and girlfriends. Women told me things such as:

- "Yeah ... I threw a glass at him. He deserved it. That'll teach him for coming home late!"
- "If I want to whip him into shape, I just tell him I'm going to call his probation officer and make up stuff. Then he really toes the line ... he does whatever I want."

- "Of course I slapped him. He was looking at the waitress when we went out to dinner. He knows better than that."

Although there were cases where women were clearly victimized, these women did not seem like powerless victims at the mercy of their abusers. In fact, if the genders had been reversed and the men had behaved as the women, each of them would have been arrested for domestic violence. In a significant number of cases, the women's behavior was even more egregious than that of their male partners.

As I worked more with men and women arrested for domestic violence, I came to recognize that this phenomenon is complex and not a "one size fits all" type of problem. The context, motivations, contributing factors, psychological issues, and relationship dynamics vary. Sometimes men truly are the dominant aggressors, and sometimes women are the dominant aggressors. Many of the men and women referred to our program are in relationships that actually are mutually abusive. In some cases, the women are the dominant aggressors, even though they are not the ones arrested, and sometimes police arrest the women when they are actually primarily victims.

Good domestic violence treatment must acknowledge these many possibilities and be tailored to the unique needs of each client. I have found that leading groups for women arrested for domestic violence is different from leading groups for men.

This book is the book I wish I had had when I first started doing groups for women.

While other programs designed for male clients may be adapted to women, this book is intentionally designed for use with women. All of the information, handouts, and role-plays are specific to women. Many examples of group situations are provided to illustrate how to deal with problems that arise. The examples are close to reality but altered to protect the anonymity of the women with whom I work.

This book is designed to provide the licensed mental health professional with a framework for understanding women's domestic violence and step-by-step direction for structuring and facilitating groups for these women. The book is divided into two parts: (1) theory and (2) practice.

In Part 1, I discuss how domestic violence is defined, the gender-inclusive perspective of domestic violence, social and cultural influences on women's violence, and how men and women are similar and different. Theories about causes of domestic violence are presented followed by discussion of effective treatment approaches and stages of change. Next, diagnostic issues and practice considerations such as safety, countertransference, cultural competence, and ethics are addressed. Part 1 concludes with information about other populations with whom this program may be useful.

While it may be tempting to skip Part 1 of this book, that will leave the therapist ill-prepared for the challenges ahead. The theory information is essential. Theory is the road map for the journey of therapy. The therapist must clearly and thoroughly understand all concepts addressed in Part 1 in order to know where her client is, where she needs to go, and how to point her in the right direction. She must be able to look behind and beyond what she sees in her clients in order to respond with the most appropriate and meaningful interventions. And her timing has to be right.

In Part 2, I provide a detailed framework for everything a therapist needs in order to set up and facilitate a domestic violence treatment program for women. Based on my experiences, I provide many examples of things that go right and how that happens, as well as things that can go wrong and options for responding therapeutically.

No single manual can provide complete guidance for every unique client and situation. Therefore, it is essential that each therapist seek regular and ongoing consultation. As we expect our clients to continue learning and growing, so must we.

I have found this work to be enormously rewarding and satisfying. I have been privileged to work with amazing women who are evidence that:

- no matter that they were never taught how to get along, how to communicate, how to negotiate in a relationship, how to share, how to resolve conflict …
- in spite of early sadness, abuse, and trauma that led them to believe they are unlovable and unworthy …
- no matter the family history of domestic violence …
- people are capable of change, capable of stopping the family patterns of hurt and sadness that are passed on generation to generation. People are capable of becoming better parents than their own and are capable of becoming better partners. People are capable of change.

Ellen L. Bowen, LCSW, BCD

Part 1

Theory

1

Understanding Domestic Violence

What Is Domestic Violence?

Domestic violence is an attempt to establish power and control in an intimate relationship (married or not, same gender or different) through the use of violence and other forms of abuse. The abuser exerts control by using physical violence, sexual violence, psychological violence, stalking, threats, harassment, intimidation, financial abuse, destruction of one's own or a partner's property, harming pets, using children to hurt a partner, identity theft, and more. Relationships involving family violence may differ in terms of the severity of the abuse, but power and control are always the underlying primary goals of all abusers.

The term *domestic violence* is often considered to include violence against children and elders, but the focus of this book is violence that occurs between intimate partners.

All 50 states have laws against domestic violence. Most focus on physical and sexual violence to the exclusion of other forms. It is important to recognize, however, that once physical or sexual violence has occurred, psychological abuse is even more powerful because the victim never knows when the abuser might be physically violent again. When a partner has been assaulted in the past, a look, a word, a threat—all carry greater power to intimidate or control.

And so, while an abuser may not actually be identified by the legal system or arrested for domestic violence, the trauma to the partner can be just as debilitating.

History of the Debate About Domestic Violence

In recent years, the field of domestic violence treatment has been filled with controversy, argument, and even acrimony over the underlying causes and responsibilities for relationship violence.

The roots of this controversy began in 1975 with the first U.S. National Family Violence Survey. In this seven-year study of over 2,000 families, Murray Strauss and Richard Gelles (1990) found that women were as violent as men.

This finding flew in the face of prevailing feminist theory, which insisted that domestic violence is rooted in patriarchy, men's use of power, male privilege, and male entitlement. Feminists argued that violent women were actually acting in self-defense, committing less serious violence, or being victims of gender-biased reporting differences. In other words, they argued that women were not really the initiators and, therefore, not really responsible for their own violence.

This debate has been fueled by two separate sets of research data. In the first, data from subsequent national surveys by Straus continued to suggest that women are as equally violent as men in intimate relationships (Straus, 1999). This was also supported by data from meta-analysis of 82 couple-conflict studies, which found that women are more likely to use physical aggression than men and resort to violence more often than men (Archer, 2000, 2002).

The opposing source of data came from the Bureau of Justice Statistics, which has consistently reported that women are five times more likely than men to have been victims of domestic violence (Rennison & Welchans, 2000).

A growing body of evidence has been found to support the existence of "husband battering" (Carney, Buttell, & Dutton, 2007). Hines, Brown, and Dunning (2003) studied calls to an American national domestic violence helpline for men. When advertised in state telephone directories, the line went from receiving 1 call per day to 250 calls per day. Nearly all callers reported physical abuse from their partners; 90% reported controlling behaviors by their partners, and 52% currently in an abusive relationship were fearful that a female partner would cause serious injury if she found out he had called the helpline. Many reported severe attacks to the groin area, stalking, and partners trying to drive over them.

Another study also strongly refuted the notion that men do not suffer harm from partner violence. In a reanalysis of the Canadian National General Social Survey (GSS) data based on a sample of 25,876, Laroche

(2005, p. 16, Table 8) concluded that victim reactions for abused men were virtually identical to those of abused women.

In a review of the literature on domestic violence research, Carney et al. (2007) concluded that while women are injured more than men, female partner violence occurs at the same rate as male partner violence. They found that women's violence tends to have a long developmental history that predates the current relationship, suggesting that it cannot be dismissed as self-defense. They also found that the most common form of partner violence is mutual, followed by female more severe and then male more severe.

The rancor that exists between opposing sides on the domestic violence debate is unfortunate in that it wastes time and resources and diverts attention from finding solutions to family violence. More and more women are being arrested for domestic violence and court-ordered to treatment (Holtzworth-Munroe, 2005). Women constitute the fastest growing segment of the criminal justice population, and the National Institute of Justice estimates that the increase in incarceration rate for women is double that of men (Ferraro & Moe, 2003; Mullings, Hartley, & Marquet, 2004).

My conviction is that if we are serious about ending domestic violence, we must be willing to address all aspects of aggression and violence in families. We must hold men *and* women accountable for their behaviors and how they choose to participate in their relationship dynamics. I believe it is time to stop arguing over who is more at fault and start looking at better ways to understand each person involved and how best to help each live safely and without violence.

Why Are Women Violent or Abusive?

Women who are abusive to their intimate partners are a heterogeneous group. They tend to fall within one of three categories:

- Dominant aggressors similar to male abusers
- Women who have fought back in self-defense but who are primarily victims of domestic violence
- Women who are in mutually aggressive relationships

While the last group is the most common, I have found that some women change from one category to another from relationship to relationship. A woman who was primarily the victim with one man may be mutually aggressive with her next partner or even be the dominant aggressor.

The reasons, motivations, context, and factors in women's violence are varied and numerous. Below we will explore several.

Underlying Beliefs

No single explanation accounts for women's violence unless it is the underlying belief that violence is an acceptable solution for women given the circumstances. Women often enter court-ordered treatment convinced that they were absolutely justified in their violence. They minimize ("All I did was throw a plate at him!"), deny ("I don't know how he tripped ... he's just clumsy"), and blame ("He made me so mad—he made me do it!").

Female Entitlement

Sometimes abusive women justify their violence by female entitlement, or female privilege. They enter romantic relationships with rigid, traditional beliefs about men's and women's roles. In their view, when a male partner has not kept his part of the bargain, they feel justified in retaliating and punishing him. Several women have told me, "We always agreed I would stay home with the kids, but now he says I have to get a job because he's leaving. I don't think so! It's his job to take care of me and pay my bills." They used this rationale to justify stalking, keeping the children away, and threatening to kill a partner.

Sociocultural Influences

Ask most people what they think of when they hear the term *domestic violence*, and invariably they will say "a man hurting a woman." Unlike men, women in our culture start from a place where they are seen as victims. Despite their childhood histories of trauma and abuse, men are never excused for hitting women. Not so with women. In fact, our culture gives them the opposite message. Women are more likely to expect that it is acceptable to hit men and that men will not retaliate.

The Double Standard

Our culture has different standards for men and women with respect to their violence. Romantic comedy movies and popular TV shows include women having temper tantrums, slapping, hitting, and assaulting men when they have been ignored, spurned, or offended. The man makes lame excuses, laughs, or runs. The audience laughs. This is entertainment. It is acceptable for women to express their rage in violent behavior because men are tough and women cannot really hurt them. But if the genders were reversed it is inconceivable that the audience would have the same response. We are conditioned to think that women's violence is funny or does not really matter.

Self-Defense

In some cases, women really are primarily the victims of domestic violence and have been arrested when they fought back. These situations can be difficult for police to evaluate, especially when the man has visible signs of injury and maintains he was innocent in the attack. Consider the woman who is being held down on the bed and choked by her husband: She uses her fingernails to claw him, leaving scratches on his arms and back. When the police respond to the neighbor's 911 call, they find marks on the husband but not the wife, so she is arrested. In another case, a man and woman are drunk and arguing in the kitchen. He grabs her in a head-lock under his arm, so she reaches for the counter, grabs a knife, and stabs him. He has a life-threatening wound, so the police arrest her.

Learned Behavior

Both men and women who are abusive with partners are likely to have grown up in families where they witnessed violence or were abused themselves.

From the beginning of our lives we all learn from what we see and experience. Our parents or other caregivers are the role models who, by their examples, teach us how to behave, how to set appropriate boundaries, how to express and cope with emotions, how to listen and how to speak, how to resolve conflict, how to love.

When our caregivers are unable to effectively manage themselves, their behavior and emotions, we do not learn how to do those for ourselves. When children see mom throw a plate of food at dad and dad retaliates by throwing mom over his knee and spanking her, they learn that this is how adults resolve their problems.

Boys and girls may identify more with the same-sex parent or with the opposite-sex parent and model their use of power and control differently.

When a father repeatedly demeans and humiliates a mother who cowers in silence, a daughter may conclude that her mother deserved it, and so does she—or she may conclude that getting what she wants in a relationship will require dominance and power over her partner.

Respectful, nurturing role models beget respect and nurturing; violent, hurtful role models beget violence and hurt.

In working with both abusive men and women, I have found that the women tend to have childhood histories that had even more trauma and instability than their male counterparts.

Mental Health Issues and Substance Abuse

In our program, about one-third of the women have histories of self-cutting or burning. Many have depression, bipolar disorder, or anxiety disorders.

According to Dutton, Nicholls, and Spidel (2005), female abusers are about as likely as male abusers to have an Axis I disorder (according to *Diagnostic and Statistical Manual of Mental Disorders* [DSM-IV] of the American Psychiatric Association), but are substantially more likely to be in the clinical range on Axis II. The personality disorder traits I see most often are those impacting intimacy, attachment, and constricted affect.

About half of the women in our program have histories of significant substance abuse. Alcohol, cocaine, and methamphetamine abuse are the most common. This makes sense considering the level of trauma they have experienced throughout childhood and adult life. They often have said that their substance use was an effort to cope with overwhelmingly painful emotions or circumstances. While they may blame their violent behavior on alcohol or drugs, we maintain that chemicals do not cause domestic violence, but they make a "good buddy" for the violence. They make violence seem like a good option.

Perceived Powerlessness

Domestic violence is often described as a phenomenon based on power and control. Abusive women and men usually feel very powerless. Both often feel threatened and defenseless, and fear abandonment. They have no ability to self-sooth and see no other options. Their violence is a desperate attempt to ward off incapacitating emotions and the accompanying perceived powerlessness.

Reasons That Abusive Women Give for Their Violence

Women give many different reasons for their violence that led them to our program, including:

- To let out anger, express feelings, release tension
- Self-defense, protection
- To feel empowered
- To get the attention of a partner, to make him listen, get him to talk
- To show him who's boss—make him do something or stop doing something
- To teach him a lesson
- To retaliate, make him hurt (e.g., for infidelity: "All those years he beat me and I stayed. When I found out he was having an affair, that was the last straw.")
- To keep him from leaving (real or perceived abandonment)
- "Just teasing"

A Final Note

A common experience is for women to be more forthcoming about their history of violence the longer they have been attending group. Many will say, "I was arrested for this one incident, but in reality I have been violent in every relationship I have ever had.... I just never got in trouble for it."

How Are Abusive Women Similar to and Different From Abusive Men?

As noted previously, female abusers share many of the same characteristics as male abusers—personality disorders, childhood experiences of witnessing domestic violence between parents, and abuse or neglect during childhood. Some significant differences also exist and can have important implications for treatment; we explore these below.

Types of Violence

While women and men initiate relationship violence at equal rates (Archer, 2000; Straus & Gelles, 1990), they tend to differ in how they are aggressive.

Men are more likely to beat up their partners, and women are more likely to hit with objects (Archer, 2002, Straus & Gelles, 1990).

My observation is that men are more likely to use physical aggression, and women are more likely to use verbal or psychological aggression. Men are more likely to punch holes in walls, and women are more likely to throw things. Men are more likely to hit, and women are more likely to slap. While he may grab her to restrain her, she is more likely to get in front of the door so he cannot leave. If he tries to control her spending, she sneaks into his wallet and takes money or runs up credit card debt.

Although the tactics are different, both sexes can use violence to exert power and control over their partners.

Communication, Personality, Social Roles, Biology

Women tend to more frequently cite emotional expression (e.g., reactive or expressive aggression: "I was just so frustrated!"), self-defense, and retaliation as reasons for their aggression. By contrast, men more frequently cite using violence in an instrumental, goal-directed manner to obtain some outcome (e.g., instrumental aggression: "I had to make her stop nagging"; Holtzworth-Munroe, 2005).

Women are more likely to place greater value on relationship intimacy and are more emotive, while men tend to value autonomy and have a more linear, problem-solving approach to relationships (Tannen, 1990). While women may be aggressive to get attention and engage their male partners, men are more likely to be aggressive to get their female partners to leave them alone (Fiebert & Gonzales, 1997).

Because of women's biology, they are uniquely affected by the physiological experiences of premenstrual syndrome, pregnancy, childbirth, postpartum depression, and the effects of these on emotions and self-care.

Personality Disorders

In a large-scale study comparing men and women arrested for domestic violence, Henning, Jones, and Holford (2003) found that while there were few demographic differences, women were about five times more likely to have elevations on a borderline scale. They also found that women were more likely to have been prescribed psychotropic medication and to have made a prior suicide attempt. These findings reflect the experiences of my clients.

History of Childhood Trauma

My experience is that women who are referred to court-mandated treatment come from even more traumatic childhood experiences than their male counterparts and have even fewer and more fragile coping skills for the most basic life challenges. Many were sexually and physically abused by a family member. Many had been in numerous foster homes where they were abused. Many had parents who forgot to feed them because of their own alcohol or drug abuse. Many witnessed domestic violence between parents, ran away from home at an early age, and dropped out of school.

The Societal Response

It is possible that the difference between men and women who are court-mandated to treatment is more a reflection of our societal reluctance to view women as domestically violent than it is a reflection of reality. One police detective told me that after investigating several cases and arresting women for domestic violence, his superior told him his statistics were off, women cannot be the primary aggressors and he needed to remember this when he was investigating these crimes.

The women referred to our program are more likely to have committed acts of greater physical violence against their partners than the referred men have. Women have stabbed, knocked unconscious, bitten off body parts, and attempted to run over their male partners. The men referred to our program are more likely to be arrested for terrorist threats (e.g., phone calls, text messages threatening to kill), pushing a partner down, grabbing her to restrain her, or pulling the phone cord out of the wall.

We know that both men and women can be violent, but perhaps it takes more incidents of violence before abusive women are arrested, prosecuted, and sentenced.

Adult History of Domestic Violence

For many women, the lines distinguishing between *abusive* and *abused* are blurred. Abusive women court-ordered to treatment present histories and symptoms more like victims of domestic violence than do their male counterparts (Abel, 1999).

Women's use of aggression can increase their risk of vulnerability to partners' aggression and risk of victimization; once violence is introduced into the relationship, male violence will have more negative effects (Bachman & Carmody, 1994; Dutton et al., 2005; Feld & Straus, 1989; Gelles & Straus, 1988; Straus, 1999).

Acting Out in Group

My own experience in working with female abusers is that compared to their male counterparts, they are infinitely more verbal and more psychologically fragile. They are more likely to view female relationships with fear and competition, and to act out in group.

For example, women have taken offense to questions posed by other group members and have retaliated with terrorist threats. One woman told another that she was having an affair with her husband and that he liked her better. When one woman was confronted about her abusive behavior toward her partner, she told the other women they had better watch their backs because she knew where they each lived.

I have never experienced these kinds of sudden, mercurial verbal assaults by any of the men with whom I have worked.

Why Don't Abused Men Report?

Powerful cultural influences inhibit men from reporting to law enforcement, family, and friends their experiences of being abused by their partners; we explore some below.

The "Wimp" Factor, the Shame of Being a Victim

In our culture, men are socialized from early childhood to suppress their emotional and physical pain. This is seen a sign of strength and manliness. Consider the playground names that boys are called if they are afraid or cry: wimp, wuss, sissy, crybaby, loser. Boys are told to "take it like a man." When they endure pain without crying, they are considered tough, macho, even heroic. Men are supposed to be self-sufficient, protective, strong.

These powerful messages from childhood tell a man that if he is hurt and complains, he is not truly a man. For the man who is being abused, the shame can be overwhelming. The greater the shame, the greater the embarrassment and the more difficult it is to tell someone else what is happening.

Our Culture Minimizes Women's Violence

Endemic to our culture is the belief that women are weaker and therefore cannot really inflict injury. It is not uncommon for men *and* women to laugh when a woman is threatening or violent and to dismiss the lethality of her behavior.

Years ago, national news reported the case of Lorena Bobbitt, who cut off the penis of her husband, John, as he slept. This story was fodder for late-night TV talk shows for many months. Although this was a horrible assault, society treated it as a joke.

If the genders were reversed and a husband cut off any part of his wife's sexual anatomy, the cultural response would be horror and outrage, not laughter.

Fear They Will Not Be Believed, Be Laughed At

A realistic fear for a male victim of domestic violence is that he will not be believed. Historically, the idea of male victimization has not been widely accepted or recognized (Straus, 1997). Because domestic violence services are so strongly biased to assume that victims are women, men seeking help may be referred to programs for male batterers (Hines et al., 2003).

Same Reasons as Women

Abused men express many of the same reasons as their female counterparts for not reporting their partners' domestic violence. They love their wives or girlfriends and want to protect them from arrest, jail, and the legal system. They promise to be more attentive and acquiescent and hope that the violence will never happen again. If they have children, they may fear for the children's safety if they report domestic violence and must leave, or worry that they will lose custody or visitation. They fear failure.

2

Theoretical Foundations for Treatment

Domestic violence occurs in all cultures, races, occupations, income levels, ages, abilities, religious preferences, and sexual orientations. No part of our society is immune.

So, if a man or a woman has a need for power and control, where does that need come from? How can power and control become such an issue in an intimate relationship that a person would resort to violence?

I believe the answers to these questions are found in a person's family of origin experience. When this history is viewed through the lens of social learning theory, attachment theory, and trauma theory, the therapist is equipped to better understand the client and more effectively help her to change.

Family of Origin

For all of us, our family of origin is the template by which we unconsciously measure our understanding of ourselves and our relationships. What our own family was like shapes how we define *family*. It is what we intuitively think of as normal because it is familiar.

If mom is often raging and dad is placating, we are more likely to experience that as normal. If dad is often raging and mom is placating, we are more likely to experience that as normal. The lessons we carry from our earliest life experiences are embedded so deeply in our memories that we often are not consciously aware of them and their power in our lives.

Through our early relationships with parents, caregivers, and siblings, we learn what acceptable behavior is for adults with adults, adults with children, and children with children. We learn what happens when the behavior is unacceptable. We learn how emotions are expressed and managed, what is talked about, and what is never discussed. We learn what is important and what is ignored. We learn what to expect in relationships:

love, trust, intimacy, respect or rejection, suspicion, distance, abuse. We learn whether or not we are important and how to get our needs met. We learn how conflicts are addressed and resolved. We learn what forgiveness is, what offenses are forgiven, and what ones can never be. We learn empathy for ourselves and for others.

The family of origin is invariably where children first learn the meaning and significance of violence. When a child is a victim of violence or witnesses parental violence, the child learns that violence is acceptable—an acceptable way to communicate and an acceptable solution for resolving problems with those you love.

Social Learning Theory

According to social learning theory, people develop behavioral habits—repeated ways of acting—by observation of role models (parents, caregivers, siblings, peers, etc.) or by self-teaching, trial and error; we learn by what we see and what works to reach our goals. We repeat behaviors that are rewarded and stop behaviors that are punished.

Parents often use a system of rewards and punishments to raise their children: treats, TV or video game time, money, privileges, or praise for good behavior, and restrictions, grounding, or reprimands for bad behavior. In school, students are rewarded for learning with good grades and punished for failing grades with having to repeat coursework. Adults are rewarded for good work performance by their paychecks and punished for poor job performance by being fired.

According to social learning theory, rewards and punishments can come in many forms. Abusive power and control can, in the moment, force someone to do what you want him to do. It can relieve tension from a stressful experience, intimidate a partner to stay in the relationship, or transform a feeling of powerlessness into a sense of omnipotence—rewards.

But abusive power and control can also challenge a partner to retaliate with greater violence. It can alienate a loved one to the point of leaving the relationship or lead to arrest, jail, restraining orders—punishments.

Social learning theory's implication and its value to treatment is this: if domestic violence is *learned*, then it can be *unlearned*. Abusive people are capable of change; they are capable of learning respectful, nonviolent ways of relating. This perspective offers hope to those who have struggled and want to do better.

On the other hand, social learning theory oversimplifies human motivations and relationships by focusing solely on responses to external stimuli. Why are some rewards and punishments effective motivators for some people and ineffective for others? How do we account for individual experience, interpretation, and choice when it comes to violent behavior? Why are some people able to resist the temptation of immediate rewards and aspire to higher moral values?

The shortcoming of social learning theory is that it ignores the existence of an "inner life," which offers other explanations for violence.

Attachment Theory

Attachment theory suggests a compelling description of inner life and how it relates to violence in intimate relationships. Based on early experiences and interactions with primary caregivers, young children develop beliefs about themselves and how their needs will be met through relationships. Different experiences create beliefs that lead to the development of different attachment styles.

The relationship a child has with her caregiver will influence the types of relationships she will have in adulthood. This theory was originally formulated by John Bowlby (1969, 1973, 1980) and expanded through the research of Mary Ainsworth et al. (1978). Cindy Hazen and Phillip Shaver (1987) and others have applied attachment theory to adult romantic relationships.

Bowlby, a British psychoanalyst, studied children (ages 15–30 months) when first separated from their caregivers (usually mothers). He observed that certain circumstances would trigger anxiety in children. They would try to alleviate this anxiety by seeking proximity and comfort from their mothers. Children went to astonishing lengths (crying, screaming, searching, clinging) to either prevent separation from their mothers or reestablish closeness after separation. He viewed this as a necessary function for survival: Young humans must depend on others for food, shelter, clothing, comfort, and security.

Bowlby maintained that if the attachment figure (mother) was nearby, accessible, and attentive, the child was more likely to feel loved, secure, and confident, allowing the child to explore the environment and play with others. If the mother was not nearby, accessible, or attentive, the child became distressed and anxious. If this continued, the child experienced rage, despair, and then detachment.

Bowlby saw anger as "protest behavior" resulting from frustrated attachment need; its purpose was to reengage a caregiver to soothe distress and anxiety when the child was not yet able to do so for herself. As such, anger was an emotion born of fear of loss. In adulthood, dysfunctional anger was defined as anger that distanced the attachment object (spouse or partner) rather than bringing him closer.

Subsequent to Bowlby's writings, Ainsworth conducted empirical research to assess infant–mother attachment in the laboratory: the strange situation. A mother brought her young child into a strange room with a few chairs and some toys on the floor. The mother was instructed to leave her child and exit the room. Ainsworth then directed a sequence of events and observed through a one-way mirror. She focused on the interaction between the child's protests and efforts to engage her mother, and the mother's responsiveness to the child's needs.

In about 70% of the mother–child dyads, Ainsworth found that mothers were attuned to their children's emotional states and responded effectively to their needs for vulnerability and independence. These mothers were able to accept their children's protests without retaliation, rejection, or anxiety. She described these children as having secure attachment.

The remaining children showed behaviors that Ainsworth viewed as defensive strategies calculated to maintain contact with rejecting or inconsistent mothers. She categorized the remaining children as exhibiting one of three types of insecure attachment styles: 15–20% insecure-avoidant, 10–15% insecure-ambivalent, and 5–10% insecure-disorganized.

The four attachment styles of childhood can be summarized as follows:

- **Secure attachment in childhood:** The child protests the mother's departure, seeks comfort, calms quickly on mother's return, accepts reassurance, and then returns to exploration (playing with toys).
- The mother is consistently responsive and accurate in reading her child's unspoken emotional cues. She picks her up and soothes her when distressed, and puts her down when she wants to go exploring. She is confident in her parenting, available, and responsive. She shows empathy and an ability to talk about emotions.
- **Insecure/avoidant attachment in childhood:** The child shows no outward signs of distress at the mother's departure and avoids eye contact upon her return. By appearing to be busy with toys, the child wards off any advances the mother may make.
- The mother appears unaware of her child's distress, is gruff when handling her child, avoids close body contact, or rebuffs the child's bids for comfort.

- **Insecure/ambivalent attachment in childhood:** The child is very distressed at the mother's departure, anxious and angry at her return, clingy and unable to let go and explore.
- The mother is significantly less attuned to her child's emotional states and unspoken needs, inconsistently responsive, more likely to ignore her child when distressed, to intrude when the child is happily playing.
- **Insecure/disorganized attachment in childhood:** The child's behavior is often extreme, vacillating between avoidant and ambivalent behavior upon mother's departure and return, showing no strategy for managing anxiety.
- Like her child, this mother shows great distress when her child is distressed, appears to have no consistent strategy for responding to her child, and no awareness of her role in her child's difficulties. She often has a childhood history of abuse or suffered a profound early loss, such as the death of a parent.

Researchers have found these same childhood attachment patterns parallel those identified in adults (Hazen & Shaver, 1987; Main, 1999).

The connection is this: Attachment is essential in life because it is how we learn to balance our need for intimacy with our need for autonomy. It is the process through which we learn to self-soothe. Through attachment to a consistent, safe, responsive adult, we feel protected in times of distress (safe harbor) and yet free to venture out and explore the world, because we have someone to lean on (secure base). We feel safe and supported.

When a caregiver is inconsistent, rejecting, shaming, or abusive, a child learns to make compromises to avoid altogether losing what little attachment she may have. Over time, she will come to believe certain things about herself and what she can expect (or not) from close relationships. She chronically searches for a secure base and feels dependent and isolated. The patterns enacted through her childhood attachments are likely the same ones she will enact in adulthood. The same concepts apply to male children as much as to female children.

The four corresponding adult attachment styles can be described as follows:

- **Secure/autonomous adult:** Most likely to describe themselves and partners in a positive light, they value attachment-related experiences, have an accurate understanding of important relationships in their lives, show compassion for others, and are able to speak coherently about how their past has influenced present feelings and relationships. They are comfortable with emotional intimacy and do not often worry about being abandoned.

- **Insecure/dismissive adult:** Having experienced close relationships as too much trouble, they appear independent to a fault, as if they do not need anyone. They tend to deny that childhood attachment experiences had any influence on their present behavior. They deal with rejection by distancing themselves and suppressing feelings. They tend to dissociate sexual from emotional commitment and are uncomfortable with emotional self-disclosure.
- **Insecure/preoccupied or ambivalent adult:** Clingy, they fall in love too easily, reveal themselves too quickly and too early in relationships, and can be excessively jealous and possessive. They often view partners as fickle and undependable. They worry that partners do not really love them or will leave.
- **Insecure/unresolved or disorganized/fearful adult:** Fearing both intimacy and abandonment, they tend to be overly demanding and angry, as well as hypersensitive to rejection. Many present with borderline personality disorder.

In her study of both partners in aggressive relationships, Bookwala (2002) examined the attachment styles of both the identified aggressors and the identified victims. She found that those with a preoccupied/ambivalent attachment style were most likely to be aggressive toward a partner. This makes sense, as this is the type most likely to experience intense anxiety about possible abandonment. When both partners had this attachment style, the likelihood of aggression was increased.

Bookwala found the strongest predictor of aggression, however, was in the combination of a partner with insecure-fearful style (uncomfortable with intimacy) and a partner with insecure-preoccupied/ambivalent style (dependent, fearing abandonment). This combination is the one I most often see in women referred to our program. An insecure, dependent woman is drawn to a distant, unreachable man. The more withdrawn he is, the more she feels abandoned and alone. She redoubles her efforts to remain connected to him. Her violence is her desperate, frantic attempt to be acknowledged, understood, and reassured.

Attachment theory has relevance not only for its explanation of the historical roots of relationship violence, but also for what it suggests for healing. An insecure attachment style can be healed through a consistent, predictable, stable relationship with a partner or through the process of psychotherapy.

Secure attachment is the essence of good therapy. The therapist provides a safe harbor and secure base for the client. The client is able to explore thoughts and feelings about childhood attachment figures and how those relate to current relationships. Through attunement experiences provided by the therapist, the client finds new ways of regulating her anxiety around abandonment or engulfment. In this process the client achieves "earned secure attachment."

Trauma and the Brain

No discussion of aggressive women would be complete without an understanding of the role of trauma in their histories. Without exception, every woman referred to our program has a significant history of trauma events that have been psychologically overwhelming and which have left her feeling especially vulnerable to real or perceived danger, mistreatment, or rejection. These events have usually included child physical or sexual abuse, witnessing domestic violence during childhood, or experiencing domestic violence from a partner.

When a person experiences a traumatic event, a cascade of stress hormones is immediately precipitated in the brain. These chemicals act on the *amygdala* and other related structures in the limbic system of the brain, which causes the heart to beat faster, blood pressure to rise, and blood glucose and insulin levels to rise, and directs blood to muscles to prepare for an emergency response to danger.

The amygdala is often referred to as being part of the reptilian or old brain, as it functions in ways we imagine to be necessary for primitive humans to survive daily life-threatening danger: A saber-toothed tiger suddenly jumps in front of you ready to devour you, and you need to be able to move fast to either fight or flee, in order to save yourself. Although none of us encounters a saber-toothed tiger nowadays, our brain retains this important stress-response survival function that is activated in other types of stressful current-day experiences.

Recent advances in brain imaging have shown that when the amygdala is activated, the prefrontal cortex is inactive. The *prefrontal cortex* is part of the new or conscious brain and is located in the area behind the forehead. It serves as the location for executive functions: perception of what is happening around us, abstract thought, formation and comprehension of language, thinking through options, and making choices. Using the saber-toothed tiger analogy, when confronted with the tiger, we do not want to stop and think about our options, we want our amygdala to take over and give us the energy surge we need to save ourselves.

It is often better to be capable of calming down and evaluating a situation before fighting or running: "Just because he'd rather watch a football game on TV, does that really mean he's bored with me? If he doesn't answer when I ask a question, does that really mean he doesn't love me, or could he be distracted or not have heard me? If he's coming home late from work and is drunk, does it mean he's been seeing someone else or could there be other explanations?"

Psychiatrist Bruce Perry (1995) maintains that throughout life, but especially during the first few years of life, the brain continues to develop and structurally organize. Repeated exposure to trauma, especially in the early years, can alter the development of the brain, leaving a person hypersensitive to threat or danger.

Trauma theory suggests that the more a person has experienced significant trauma—whether attachment trauma or physical, sexual, or emotional abuse—the greater the likelihood she will experience either immediate or lasting symptoms. Common immediate responses include dissociation; Stockholm syndrome, where a victim becomes attached or bonded to a perpetrator; learned helplessness (Walker, 1984); and relief at surviving, yet also guilt. Longer lasting responses to trauma include substance abuse, panic attacks, flashbacks, experiencing relationships as dangerous, expecting to be criticized, humiliated, misunderstood, laughed at, hurt, retraumatized, and so forth (Briere & Scott, 2006).

For some, it is as if their amygdalas are stuck in a permanently on position, ready to fight or flee, with no access to logical thoughts that might help them calm, self-soothe, or think things through. Violence is, in a sense, a desperate, primitive attempt to defend against painful affects such as fear, grief, abandonment, or powerlessness reminiscent of past painful or traumatic experiences.

The core experiences of trauma are disempowerment and disconnection from others. Recovery happens as the survivor is empowered in her life and is able to create new connections to others. Healing from trauma can only occur in the context of relationships.

3

Effective Treatment

The value in understanding these different theoretical perspectives is that they reflect the diversity in women who come to treatment. They underscore the notion that one size does *not* fit all.

It is essential that the therapist avoid personal biases and preconceived ideas about violent women. Some women have been primarily victimized throughout childhood but not in adult relationships, some were not abused in childhood but have been abused in adult relationships, some are primarily the aggressors, and many present as a complex mix where the lines of distinction between victim and aggressor are blurred. Some have psychiatric disorders and many do not. Some women enter treatment enraged at the legal system, resistant to examining their own behavior, while others are more repentant and eager to learn and change.

Effective treatment takes into consideration this diversity as well as women's varying and shifting levels of motivation for change.

Stages of Change and Motivational Interviewing

A helpful way of conceptualizing readiness for change is offered by the transtheoretical model and motivational interviewing (Prochaska et al., 1992). Originally used to understand how people overcome health-related problems such as smoking, obesity, lack of exercise, and alcohol and drug addiction, this model is also helpful in conceptualizing how abusive women change.

In this model, a person who is trying to change a behavior must go through a progression of stages in order to make the change. Moving through the stages requires effort, energy, planning, and follow-through. The earlier stages of commitment and motivation are essential for the later stages of actually changing behavior. Motivational interviewing is used to promote movement from one stage to the next. The stages of change are as follows:

1. **Precontemplation:** "I don't have a problem with violence, I have no interest in changing my behavior."
2. **Contemplation:** "I am realizing that I do have a problem with violence, but I'm not sure I want to do anything about it yet ... maybe later."
3. **Preparation:** "Not only do I recognize that I have a problem with violence, but I really want to do something about it so that my future will be better."
4. **Action:** "My past violence is unacceptable. I am taking steps every day to do things differently and to practice new skills I am learning. I ask for advice and follow through with it. I am motivated to make myself better because I want it—not just because the judicial system is telling me I have to. I am committed to change."
5. **Maintenance:** "While I am continuing to change, I recognize I need to continue being consistent and vigilant. This is a lifelong process. I choose friends, work, and leisure activities that support and reinforce my commitment to nonviolence in my relationships. If I get stuck or see early warning signs of old behaviors, I acknowledge them and do whatever I can to seek help so that I don't return to how I used to be."

What traditional psychotherapy may label as resistance or denial, motivational interviewing views as a normal stage in the process of change. It is seen as an indication that a person has not yet perceived the importance of change or has not yet recognized a large enough discrepancy between her current status and her desired, expected ideal. Good treatment matches interventions to a client's particular stage of change and motivates her to continue to the next stage.

For example, when women have been court-ordered to domestic violence treatment, they are often in the precontemplative stage of change: they think they have no problems or issues requiring counseling and instead focus on how angry they are with the legal system and how they feel unfairly punished. Arguing with them is fruitless and countertherapeutic because it establishes an adversarial relationship.

Motivational interviewing views treatment as a process of collaboration with the client. The aim is to draw out the client's own perceptions, goals, and values and affirm her capacity for self-direction. The therapist is empathic and accepting. The client's ambivalence is viewed as normal. The therapist motivates the client to consider change by pointing out the discrepancy between her current behavior and her stated goals or values. "I can see that you really care about your boyfriend. He means the world to you. But it seems that calling him names and threatening to kill him doesn't match up with who you are or the love you tell me you feel toward him."

If the client disputes the suggestion of discrepancy, the therapist does not argue for change. Resistance is viewed as a signal to respond differently. The client is the primary source for new answers and solutions. Her belief in the possibility of change is an important motivator. The client—not the counselor—is responsible for choosing and carrying out change. When this happens, the counselor's belief in the person's ability to change becomes a self-fulfilling prophecy.

Through the course of treatment, the therapist matches interventions to the client's stage of change. For example, when a woman is in the pre-contemplative stage, the therapist does not lecture but instead facilitates the client's assessment of her particular situation—the pros and cons of changing or even of making a decision to change. By being nonthreatening and supportive, the therapist encourages the client to take responsibility for her own situation.

The therapist's role transitions from motivating to advising or coaching when the client decides to change. The therapist helps the client anticipate obstacles, identifying possible support systems, reinforcing accomplishments, and affirming self-efficacy.

Treatment Goals

The program outlined in this book is designed to address topics as required in the domestic violence laws of the State of California. Other state laws have similar requirements. The approach is psychoeducational and psychotherapeutic. Specific skills taught include healthy communication, cooldowns and time-outs, assertiveness, empathy, and attunement. In addition, opportunity is provided for deeper healing from childhood and adult trauma. My conviction is that through healing these deeper psychological wounds, a woman will be better equipped to sustain positive changes, to relate nonviolently with her partner and her children, and to become a happier, more productive person.

Drawing on the various perspectives previously discussed, the treatment goals are for a client to

1. Stop violent behavior.
2. Take responsibility for her own violent and abusive behavior without minimizing, blame, or denial.
3. Identify physical, emotional, and behavioral cues that signal escalating danger. (This does not mean placating a partner on every issue, but rather being aware of her own as well as her partner's responses to conflict and taking responsibility for her own.)
4. Establish safety—both physical and emotional—for herself, her children, and her partner.
5. Understand the dynamics and effects of domestic violence. Identify unhealthy and abusive interaction patterns, compared to healthy and nonabusive interaction patterns.
6. Learn skills for respectful communication, problem solving, and conflict resolution with a partner as well as with her children.
7. Learn skills to respond effectively to daily life stressors.
8. Learn emotional self-regulation; increase capacity to tolerate and internally reduce painful emotional states.
9. Overcome the effects of childhood or adult trauma so that the traumatic memory is transformed and integrated into a survivor's life story.
10. Increase capacity for empathy and compassion for self and others.
11. Increase autonomy and self-esteem.

Not all women who enter this type of program will be able to attain all of these goals in 52 weeks of group treatment. The first four goals are mandatory for all participants to achieve. Goals 5–8 speak to basic relationship and life skills that will help them attain the first three goals. Goals 9–11 will give them the greatest chance for success in maintaining all of the changes spoken of in the previous goals.

For many, violence has been a lifelong response to unhappiness and a deep-rooted pattern. This program represents for them the beginning of a journey of change; they will benefit most from moving on to individual or couples therapy.

Role of the Therapist: Balancing Compassion and Support With Accountability

Successful progress in treatment depends on a positive therapeutic alliance that is based on empathy and attunement from the very beginning. With this, the client can feel understood, seen, and cared for, and thereby experience greater motivation to change. Without this, the client will not trust the therapist, will not feel safe, and will not self-disclose—essential elements of the therapeutic process.

In many ways, being a good therapist is like being a good parent, balancing two very different and seemly opposing roles. The therapist must balance compassion and support with accountability. The therapist must provide a safe harbor for the client to experience and examine emotions, providing support and compassion for the pain she has experienced that has led to her abusive behaviors. At the same time, the therapist must also hold the client fully responsible for her behaviors and choices, at times confronting and setting appropriate limits. In this, the therapist acts as an external regulator—modeling emotional literacy, helping the client to develop self-awareness and new narratives that ultimately allow hope.

A final note: Clearly not all therapists are cut out to work with abusive women. We need to be honest with ourselves about what we can and cannot tolerate because the stories we must listen to, witness, and hold will most certainly elicit our own intense feelings and pain. Through this process, we will have to examine ourselves, our own fears and insecurities, families of origin, life experiences, love relationships, reasons for doing this work, and preconceived prejudices about working with this population. When we put together our program, I wondered if I would be angry with our clients or afraid of them. I have been a clinical social worker for 35 years and I now know that I could not have done this work when I was younger. It has taken seasoning and maturing life experiences to help me understand.

4

Diagnostic Issues and Categories

As noted earlier, women who are violent toward intimate partners defy simple classification. Thorough assessment is critical in order to understand the unique history, qualities, and motives for violence of each woman. It is important that the therapist maintain an open mind and not make assumptions about these women, as it is unlikely that one diagnosis will accurately fit each woman referred for treatment.

Domestic violence, per se, is not a diagnosis but rather a description of behavior. Some women will have no diagnosis on Axis I, II, or III using the Multiaxial Assessment detailed in the American Psychiatric Association's (2000) *Diagnostic and Statistical Manual of Mental Disorders* (DSM-IV). Most, however, will have diagnoses recorded on Axis I or II—either substance abuse disorders, affective disorders, personality disorders, or medical conditions (especially those related to menstrual cycle problems, pregnancy, abortion, miscarriage, childbirth, etc.)

This chapter will focus on three general areas important in formulating a diagnostic picture of a woman referred for domestic violence treatment:

- The category or type of partner violence
- Substance abuse issues
- Psychiatric disorders

Category or Type of Partner Violence

Domestic violence, whether female perpetrated or male perpetrated, can be conceptualized as a phenomenon that occurs on a continuum and from different perspectives:

Once ... Occasionally ... Frequently
Unilateral ... Mutual
Expressive ... Instrumental
Situational Couple Violence ... Coercive/Controlling (Intimate Terrorism)

In each case, the domestic violence must be understood in context of the relationship. A woman may be the primary aggressor, equally abusive as her partner, or primarily the victim—or somewhere in between.

Her violence may be primarily a function of her poor impulse control and dysfunctional communication skills (expressive violence). Or it may be a function of her efforts to dominate and control her partner (instrumental violence). She may be the primary initiator of violence or use violence to resist the violent and controlling behavior of her partner.

Both partners' behavior may be violent but not highly controlling (situational couple violence). In these cases, violence is precipitated by conflict in the relationship.

Or one partner (or both) may be severely violent and highly controlling, as in coercive-controlling violence or intimate terrorism. These represent a minority of domestic violence cases. The offender uses fear, intimidation, harassment, and threats to coerce the victim into submission.

Substance Abuse Issues

While not all abusive women have problems with substance abuse, many do. For many, alcohol or drug use (by them or their partners) is a significant contributor to the violence. When a partner abuses alcohol or drugs, it is much easier for a woman to also do so. It is also easier for her to minimize or deny the impact on her judgment and behavior or blame her partner and *his* substance abuse.

Each woman should be assessed on an individual basis with regard to her need for concurrent substance abuse treatment while in a domestic violence treatment program. Some women will first need residential treatment to withdraw or detox from substances, while for others, outpatient treatment will be adequate.

My experience is that the most common substances abused by violent women are alcohol and methamphetamine (meth).

Alcohol

As a mood-altering chemical, alcohol is legal, socially acceptable, and readily available. It is easy to abuse, especially if a woman is already unhappy with herself or her life. Diagnostic distinction is made between alcohol abuse (use causing impairment and distress) and alcohol dependence (continued use despite consequences, including cravings, loss of control, physical dependence, and increased tolerance.)

A quick tool for screening for alcohol problems is the CAGE questionnaire (Ewing, 1984):

1. Have you ever felt the need to Cut down on alcohol consumption?
2. Are you Annoyed when people question your drinking habits?
3. Do you feel Guilty about your alcohol use?
4. Have you ever used alcohol as an Eye opener to recover from a hangover?

This questionnaire is intended to provide only guidelines, not diagnostic criteria. Answering yes to any one question suggests a possible alcohol problem. Answering yes to two or more indicates a high risk of alcohol abuse or dependence.

Methamphetamine

While women abuse the same drugs that men do, meth has a special allure for women over other drugs (California Department of Alcohol and Drug Programs [CDADP], 2007). It reduces appetite, produces rapid and dramatic weight loss, enhances mood, increases energy, and reduces fatigue. Meth can provide an escape from painful feelings—especially those associated with trauma, violence, and abuse. Meth is often introduced by a boyfriend or husband (who is also using it) as a way to have fun together and increase sexual pleasure.

On the negative side, meth is highly addictive. Long-term use leads to severe damage to teeth, badly scarred skin from compulsive scratching, insomnia and sleep disturbance, psychosis, anxiety, paranoia, depression, and hopelessness. Meth-induced paranoia can create suspicion and accusations, increasing the likelihood of domestic violence.

A woman using meth is unable to function adequately as a parent. Besides the paranoia, anxiety, and irritability, she likely pays little attention to her children's basic needs for food, sleep, hygiene, and basic well-being.

Meth use has important implications for treatment because it results in significant injury to the brain. Meth affects areas that control memory, judgment, impulse control, and mood states. During early months of recovery, symptoms may actually worsen before they improve. Memory is poor but recovers in the first few weeks of abstinence. Sleep and dream states are typically disrupted for several months. Addicts often experience anhedonia (inability to experience pleasure) for six months and may question whether recovery is worth it.

Because of the dramatic brain damage that meth brings, it is imperative that a woman with any history of meth use be abstinent before entering a domestic violence treatment program. The necessary length of abstinence may vary and should be determined by the therapist on a case-by-case basis.

However, it is important for the therapist to remember that the woman's ability to remember basic information will be impaired for a while. Information should be presented in a simple and straightforward way and repeated often. It is also important to reassure the addict that the longer she is abstinent, the more things will improve.

Psychiatric Disorders

While not all violent women have psychiatric disorders, many do. My experience is that the most common are the Cluster B Personality Disorders and disorders related to history of traumas. DSM-IV details the criteria for these disorders. In short, they are as follows:

- Adjustment disorder
- Acute stress disorder
- Posttraumatic stress disorder

In some cases, women will benefit from psychotropic medication to help with symptoms of anxiety and depression. Some may also need ancillary therapy outside of group.

Cluster B Character Disorders

- **Antisocial personality disorder:** Pattern of disregard for the rights of others. "Rules aren't meant for me—only for other people. If other people are offended or hurt by my behavior, that's their problem. I will do whatever I want to get whatever I want."
- **Narcissistic personality disorder:** Pattern of grandiosity, need for admiration, lack empathy. "I am better than anyone else. I deserve special rules and consideration. I shouldn't have to interact with people who are not like me. No one should have more of anything than I have. I must always have my way."
- **Histrionic personality disorder:** Pattern of excessive emotionality and attention seeking. "Appearances—especially beauty—are most important. Emotions should always be expressed—quickly, directly, dramatically. Others exist to serve and admire me. I must be noticed."
- **Borderline personality disorder:** Pattern of instability in interpersonal relationships, self-image, and affects. Marked impulsivity. "I am not sure who I am. My emotional pain is so great it is intolerable. My feelings control me. Others are either so good that I am very lucky, or so bad that I can't stand them. I will eventually be abandoned."

Common to anyone with a character disorder is that she tends to view her problems as resulting from the environment (other people, other circumstances) rather than because of who she is, how she behaves, and how she treats others.

Because character disorders describe a person's core traits, which are inflexible and damaging, they may be seen as incurable. While they may not be able to be "cured," people with personality disorders can become higher functioning with treatment for attitude and behavioral changes.

5

Practice Issues, Cultural Competence, Ethical Considerations

Practice Issues

Safety

As has been reiterated throughout this book, safety for all must be the cornerstone of any domestic violence treatment program.

Questions for the therapist to consider are: Do I feel safe in my office space and building? How will women enter and exit the group room? With whom might they cross paths? How can we make this office environment more respectful of confidentiality so that clients can feel emotionally safe? What can we do to make our office more safety conscious? What is our plan in case of emergency (fire, earthquake, intruder, etc.)? Is there a landline phone in the group room?

Transference and Countertransference

Working with this population is an intense clinical experience that may arouse strong emotions in the therapist as well as in clients. It is essential that the therapist maintain clear and firm internal and external boundaries. She must remain consciously aware of the lines between her own feelings and projections onto the group members, and vice versa.

Whatever the therapist's family of origin experiences, she may have flashbacks that remind her of painful times when she felt abandoned, powerless, shamed, or full of rage. While group is not the appropriate setting for her to resolve these feelings, her own countertransference may provide her with helpful information to understand her clients' struggles.

In those cases, she becomes "the good momma"—a caring adult who understands, acknowledges feelings, comforts, sets limits, and holds a client accountable for her behavior. At its best, this is a powerful, reparative experience for the client.

When the emotions elicited within the therapist are overwhelming, it is important that she recognize this and seek her own therapy. This is difficult work. Not everyone is ready to do this.

By the same token, clients are likely to have their own transference toward the therapist. Those with histories of abuse and trauma may relate to the therapist as a representation of the adult who abused them or the adult who should have protected them but did not. The therapist must remain grounded and calm during these circumstances in order to effectively help them process and understand their feelings.

Caution About Concurrent Couples Therapy or Family Therapy

Many states, including California, prohibit a person court-ordered to domestic violence treatment from participating in couples therapy or family therapy until completion of the required program. The rationale for this is based on the concern that if the offender has not adequately taken responsibility for his or her violent behavior and learned anger management skills, then victims are at greater risk of being blamed or reviolated.

When concurrent couples or family therapy is not prohibited by law, I believe that these may be very helpful. Often, partners remain together and even live in the same home following a domestic violence incident. Under the right circumstances, families may more quickly resolve problems and heal from past trauma when allowed these options.

When state law allows, decisions for concurrent therapy should be based on the offender's acceptance of responsibility for her or his violent behavior, the desire and willingness of both partners to participate, and the assessment by involved therapists that this will not create a greater risk to safety for anyone in the family.

Cultural Competence

Cultural competence is essential for every therapist and begins with the recognition of one's own racial awareness and racial sensitivity. Race and racism have a profound effect on our daily lives. Whether individual or institutional, overt or covert, intentional or unintentional, there are a variety of ways in which racism can penetrate the therapy process.

Racial awareness is the ability to recognize that race exists and that it shapes reality in inequitable and unjust ways. Racial sensitivity is the capacity to anticipate how others may think and feel racially, and to adjust and accommodate one's own behaviors accordingly. This requires empathy—the ability to relate in ways that make others feel racially understood and comfortable.

Ethnic and cultural backgrounds pervade every aspect of how we view domestic violence:

- What we define as acceptable and what we define as abusive
- The abuser's tactics
- The victim's coping strategies
- The community and institutional responses
- The quality of the therapist-client relationship

Therefore, it is imperative that the therapist recognize that her worldview and experiences are likely very different from those of clients of a different race or culture.

Because most people of color have had extensive exposure to whites, they often learn from an early age how to relate to whites in ways to make them feel comfortable. In contrast, many whites lack racial sensitivity during cross-racial interactions.

A first step toward cultural competence is to explore one's own racial identity. Questions to consider are:

- How do I define myself racially?
- When did I first become aware of race or skin color?
- What messages have I received about race or skin color? From my family? From friends? From the media?
- How did those messages influence my feelings about myself?
- What benefit have I gained because of race or skin color?
- Have I ever dated a person of another race or skin color? Why or why not?

Cultural competence means recognizing that race, racism, or culture may be a part of the presenting problem. It means the therapist is sensitive to the ways in which these factors may shape clients' reality.

When a client believes that these factors are pertinent to her problems, it is important to validate her perspective, even when the therapist does not agree. The therapist acknowledges how difficult it is for the client and invites her to share examples of when she felt racially or cultural mistreated, asking: "How did this make you feel? What did you do with these feelings? Did you tell anyone else what happened? Do you feel like there is anyone else who understands what you are going through?"

The goal is to deepen the discussion and help the client consider not only the other person's contribution to the problem, but also the her own contribution.

Any time a group member makes a racially hostile or insensitive remark toward the therapist, group members, partners, or others, this must be acknowledged and challenged. When a therapist ignores such a remark, she unwittingly colludes with the racism. Sometimes she may choose to simply state that a remark is racist and, therefore, disrespectful and inappropriate. Usually, however, it will be more helpful to the learning experience of all to ask the woman to explore in group her beliefs and biases about race and culture. This can then be used as a springboard for the whole group to discuss racism.

Because many communities have people of varying racial and cultural backgrounds, it may be difficult for the well-intentioned therapist to be knowledgeable about each. What she can do, however, is acknowledge what she does not know and invite the client to educate her.

Ethical Considerations

A therapist's strong sense of integrity and ethics is essential when working with anyone, but especially with clients who have every reason to be mistrustful of a therapist whom they are ordered to see.

The forms provided later in this book provide some definition of the ethical responsibilities of the therapist. Many additional confounding circumstances can arise through the course of therapy that require that the therapist have very clear personal and professional boundaries. Consultation with seasoned colleagues, ethics committees of professional organizations, and attorneys can provide more clear direction in these situations.

In addition to meeting the local or state requirements to provide domestic violence treatment for court-ordered offenders, the therapist should

- Hold a license to practice psychotherapy
- Belong to a professional organization and abide by its code of ethics (i.e., California Society for Clinical Social Work, American Board of Examiners in Clinical Social Work, Center for Clinical Social Work, National Association of Social Workers, California Association of Marriage and Family Therapists, American Psychological Association, American Psychiatric Association)
- Maintain malpractice insurance
- Seek regular clinical consultation from colleagues
- Maintain clinical records that document all aspects of treatment
- Continue to obtain continuing education related to domestic violence, relationships, cultural competency, ethics, and so forth
- Seek legal consultation (with an attorney who specializes in legal issues related to therapy)—especially with questions regarding confidentiality, privilege, subpoenas for records or to testify in court, duty to warn, ethics, and so forth

Even for the solo group therapist, this work should not be done alone. The most effective treatment occurs when the therapist continues to seek education, consultation, and collaboration with other community colleagues.

6
Use of This Therapy With Other Groups

Individual Therapy for Women

Domestic violence treatment is most powerful and transforming when accomplished in a group setting. The group acts as a representation of the society at-large and redefines for each member the cultural norms of respect and nonviolence. This happens in a way that may not occur as effectively for the court-ordered, reluctant client in individual therapy.

In some cases, however, group therapy either is not an option or is not a viable treatment choice, for example, when:

- The woman's mental health problems are so serious as to make a group setting too distressful for her to benefit and learn
- The woman's behavior is so disruptive or inappropriate that it interferes with the therapeutic experience of the other group members

Care must be taken to ensure the confidential safety of the group. If a woman is referred who has a relative or former rival in the current group, then she should be referred to a different program, placed in a different group, or provided individual therapy.

Smaller communities may not have many treatment options. Ideally, a woman who is connected to a current group member will be treated by a different therapist than that of her relative or rival. These clients typically already have difficulty enough with trust. Discovering that they share the same therapist as someone else with whom they have had a conflicted relationship can reinforce suspicion and derail the entire treatment.

In all of these cases, a woman may be seen in individual therapy in lieu of group treatment.

Male Offenders

This program is generally appropriate for use with men who have been abusive. Handouts written to a female perspective would need to be reworded for the male perspective.

My experience is that men are very responsive to addressing family of origin issues and understanding how their childhood experiences have shaped them. Because men may be abused as well as abusive, it is important for them to understand their responsibility for their own and their children's safety.

Adolescents

Clients often tell us: "I wish I had known this when I was a teenager!" or "This should be taught in school." The recognition is that the sooner people are able to learn about healthy relationships, the better. I absolutely agree with this.

In our community we are finding more and more juveniles are being arrested for violence and court-ordered to treatment. Many are in trouble for aggression at school, at home, and in relationships with peers or romantic partners.

This program is appropriate for this age group, but with some modifications. If the juvenile is not an emancipated minor, treatment forms will need to include consent for treatment by the parent or guardian. Because relationships, love, expression of emotions, and aggression are learned at home, it is important that parents and guardians understand the principles of the program, strongly support the adolescent's participation, and commit to addressing their own problems. A family interview can serve as a helpful initial assessment with recommendations for concurrent therapy for parents as appropriate.

Lesbian, Gay, Bisexual, Transgender (LGBT) Clients

While lesbian, gay, bisexual, and transgender people are abusive toward partners at the same rate and for the same reasons as their straight counterparts, additional factors must be considered in planning effective treatment for them.

Some therapists automatically place LGBT clients in their heterosexual domestic violence treatment groups, but I strongly believe this is an insensitive mistake. Placement should be considered on a case-by-case basis, and ideally, a program should offer a separate group for LGBT clients as a treatment option.

If the therapist is not a member of this community, it is critical that she be educated about the unique needs and special concerns of this population.

She must examine her personal and clinical biases and assumptions. What other experiences has she had interacting with LGBT people? What were the experiences like? What emotions did she have? Did she question her sexual orientation or feel uncomfortable? How did she deal with that? If she has had little or no experience with any LGBT people, why not? Are any of her friends or family members LGBT? How have those around her reacted to them? How and when did she realize she is heterosexual? Does she secretly believe that homosexuality is really caused by childhood trauma or deep-seated family dysfunction? Is she able to recognize limitations in her attitudes, beliefs, and knowledge and seek consultation?

Assuming that sexual orientation has nothing to do with domestic violence can be as erroneous as assuming it is the central cause for domestic violence. Consider the following:

Cultural oppression: Our culture is rife with myths and stereotypes about homosexuality. LGBT clients are likely to already have experienced high rates of homophobic abuse—both psychological and physical—at school, home, church, and work. Because of cultural oppression, they are at greater risk for depression and anxiety.

Internalized homophobia: Discrimination suffered by LGBT people is often internalized, creating stress, low self-esteem, and difficulty establishing committed relationships.

Heterosexual privilege: LGBT couples and families lack legal legitimacy and societal validation of their relationships. Even when laws use gender-neutral terms, they are often applied inconsistently in acknowledging, protecting, or defending LGBT people. In most areas, LGBT couples are unable to marry even though they have a lifetime commitment to one another and co-parent their children. LGBT people have few positive media images or role models. This makes it difficult for them to have internalized models for healthy partnerships. Because domestic violence is thought of as a heterosexual problem, they may not realize they are experiencing it or may blame themselves.

Reluctance to report domestic violence: If an LGBT client has worked hard for acceptance and validation by her family of origin, she may be even more reticent to disclose domestic violence within her relationship and seek support from her family. Because this population is so marginalized by society, many view their LGBT community as a safe haven from violence and abuse. Intimate partners tend to be more dependent on each other ("it's us against the outside world"). They sometimes describe the fear that they are betraying their "own" by reporting domestic violence.

What if a partner is not "out?" Threatening to out a partner to family, employers, neighbors, or ex-spouse is a reprehensible and intimidating means of exerting power and control in an LGBT relationship. Consider the teacher who risks losing her job because of community fears that homosexuality corrupts children, the clergyperson whose denomination preaches that homosexuality is sin, the officer who wants a military career and knows she faces immediate discharge if her orientation is disclosed. This aspect of domestic violence is unique to the LGBT couple and leaves the victim feeling confused, ashamed, and embarrassed.

Challenges to safety and help seeking: Both LGBT abusers and victims face barriers to receiving help. The vast majority of shelters are designed exclusively for heterosexual women. Staff members are often inadequately trained to address the special needs of LGBT clients and have difficulty differentiating between abuser and victim. If a female victim escapes to a battered women's shelter, she risks her abusive female partner obtaining access to the shelter by claiming she, too, was abused.

Recommendations: If a client is referred by a probation officer or the court, the therapist should be given information that would suggest sexual orientation and gender identity. The therapist should allow the person to self-identify. Ask what the person would like to be called (he/she) even if the gender appears different or obvious. Then, use whatever pronouns are requested.

Consider: What does the client want? Is she out to family, friends, coworkers, the community? Will she be likely to feel safe in the group, able to open up and communicate any negative feelings or misunderstandings she may experience from the therapist and group members? How does she want to be referred to in group, and how does she want her partner or her relationship characterized?

If the therapist is uncertain or has questions, it is best to acknowledge this and invite the client to educate her.

Part 2

Practice

7

Before Group
Setting the Stage for Change to Occur

Thoughtful planning before starting a group helps the therapist feel more prepared and increases the likelihood of therapeutic success in the group. This chapter describes preliminary groundwork and possible obstacles and options for addressing them before a client starts in the group.

Ideally, the group therapist not only is a licensed clinician but also has significant experience working with diverse populations and a variety of presenting problems. The more clinical and life experience, the better, as clients will more likely see her as a wise, helpful resource. In this case, a single therapist can competently facilitate this type of group.

If, however, the therapist is a novice or has never facilitated groups, it is prudent to co-facilitate the group with a more experienced clinician. Many prefer to co-lead with a female–male team. This offers the advantage of modeling appropriate, respectful, egalitarian interactions between men and women. It allows for a sharing of treatment perspectives and can enrich the experience of group members. But it also requires that the therapists have mutual respect for one another professionally and an ability to work collegially. Much like what happens in a family, group members will be keenly alert to any overt conflict as well as unspoken tension between therapists and may respond with heightened anxiety, triangulation, withdrawal, or acting out in group. Co-therapists must be alert to these possibilities and allow time outside of group to discuss their own professional relationship as well as find ways to make their experiences positive learning opportunities for group members.

This book is written as if the group is facilitated by a single therapist. Co-therapists can easily follow the format, choosing how they will divide and share various responsibilities. It is essential, however, that both therapists be present for each assessment interview and preferably for each group meeting. They are each establishing a separate relationship and, together, a conjoint relationship with each client. It is critically important that they share with each other any separate interaction with clients.

While some women may enter group on their own, most, at least initially, will be referred by either the court or a probation officer. The value of a strong, collaborative working relationship with referring judges and probation officers cannot be stressed enough. Probation officers typically ensure that probationers comply with the terms set by the judge when they were placed on probation following a guilty verdict: attendance and participation in a domestic violence treatment program, community service, payment of fines, chemical testing to ensure that the probationer is free of alcohol and drugs, and unannounced home visits to ensure that she has no weapons. As law enforcement officers, probation officers act as a liaison with the court. They can provide the therapist with helpful background information about a client, such as criminal history, substance abuse history, education, vocational history, summary of the domestic violence incident and disposition, prior incidents of violence, treatment history, and assessment of risk of lethality. When this information is provided before the assessment interview, the therapist is better equipped to ascertain the client's degree of truthfulness or denial. Ongoing collaboration will improve both the therapist's and the court's understanding of a client and better facilitate her progress.

Developing the Therapeutic Alliance

In reading through the forms that a client must agree to in order to be accepted into the program, it is clear that there are a lot of rules: attendance, participation, homework, as well as rules about tardiness, absences, sobriety, and so forth. In addition, clients are told that their compliance with rules and quality of participation in the program will be regularly reported to probation and the court. Compliance with these different requirements often reflects motivation.

For a woman who has been arrested, jailed, and tried and convicted of domestic violence, this level of structure can seem intimidating and even impossible. This is especially true if she has also been abused by a partner or if she has been separated from her children because of her own violence. She is likely to contact a program with trepidation, under duress, and to see treatment as further punishment. The therapist need not argue this perspective, only recognize that it is valid in the client's eyes.

Structure and boundaries help communicate that she is expected to take the program seriously. Consistent, predictable structure maximizes the potential for each woman to feel safe disclosing about herself in group, which in turn empowers her to benefit most from the program. Clients have a right to learn and grow, and the therapist has a right to facilitate this process.

Trial and error has led our program to follow the assessment procedures described in the rest of this chapter. In the end, we found these to be the most efficient use of time. Information is repeated on the phone, verbally in person, and in written paperwork. Appointments are scheduled only when the client is ready to proceed.

A significant advantage of this early process is that a woman's response is often an indicator of areas she may have difficulty complying with when she is attending group. If she waits to the last minute to contact the program, tries to negotiate away the assessment fees, is late to the brief initial appointment or to the assessment interview, or does not have the paperwork read and completed, she is more likely to be late to group, not have homework completed, or to fall behind in fee payments.

An important note about language: Vocabulary and terminology matter. While a program may be certified under state law as a batterer intervention program, the terms *batterer*, *abuser*, and *offender* are often experienced as emotionally or politically charged for women. Words that shame a woman who has been violent to someone she loves are ultimately countertherapeutic.

A more helpful perspective communicates the message that she is at her core *a good person* who has *behaved badly*. And so, a woman is referred to as a client, participant, or group member. Because she may also have been abused by her boyfriend or husband, rather than referring to him as the victim, he is referred to as her partner. In addition, many participants refer to the program as a life skills and relationship skills class, rather than a batterer intervention program or therapy.

The First Contact

The therapeutic relationship begins with the first contact, the first phone call. This first impression sets the tone for what the woman expects in how she will be treated by the therapist as their relationship develops. Will she be treated with compassion and respect? Harshness or shame? Will she be viewed as human and therefore worthy, or as a criminal, incapable of change?

Some programs or agencies have a secretary respond to initial phone calls, explain the program requirements, conduct a brief screening, and schedule assessment appointments with the therapist. I believe this is a poor plan and compromises the development of the therapeutic alliance. The sooner the client is interacting with the therapist—on all matters— the better. Ambivalence about treatment is often expressed through complaints about fees, rules, the judge, and so forth. When the therapist is able to address these concerns from the beginning, she is able to more effectively respond to underlying ambivalence and fears about treatment.

The woman has usually been directed by the probation officer to call the program, usually by a certain date. Bearing in mind all of the information already discussed, a prompt (same day) return of her phone message communicates professionalism, responsiveness, caring, and accessibility by the therapist.

The therapist introduces herself and asks for the woman's name, address, phone numbers, probation officer's name, and next court review date. (The latter is significant because it may reflect the woman's motivation for the program: Women who wait to call until the day before their next hearing before the judge tend to be more ambivalent about participating in a treatment program.)

This initial phone contact is also the time to inform the woman of when the group meets, in case it conflicts with her work schedule or child care needs. The therapist then describes the process for assessment and acceptance into the program:

- The first step for the woman is to pay the *assessment fee*, which covers the cost of the assessment interview. This amount is fixed and must be paid in cash or money order—no personal checks (bounced checks create bookkeeping nightmares). Requiring that this fee be paid *before* the assessment interview is scheduled will significantly decrease no-shows.
- When the woman has the money for the assessment fee, she is given a five-minute appointment to meet with the therapist to:
  - Pay the assessment fee
  - Receive an appointment to return at a later date for the assessment interview (which takes one hour)
  - Receive a packet of paperwork that she must complete and bring back with her to the assessment interview
- This assessment fee is nonrefundable. If she does not show for the assessment interview, is late, or does not have the paperwork read and com-

pleted, the interview will be cancelled and she must begin the process again (paying the assessment fee before another interview is scheduled).

- It is important to explain to the woman that just because she has made this phone call does not mean she is accepted into the program. She still must be assessed and accepted in order to be enrolled.

What if she objects?

- "Oh that's just great! All I'm doing is getting punished!" The therapist may respond: "You are right, there are a lot of rules. It can seem pretty overwhelming at the beginning. Would you like to think about it and call me later when you are ready to proceed?"
- "I'm only doing this because I don't want to go back to jail." The therapist may respond: "Staying out of jail is a good goal to have," and then ask about other motivating factors for her staying out of jail, for example, children, partner, job, school.
- "I can't believe I have to pay for this! What a rip-off!" The therapist may respond: "Yes, you do have to pay for this and it adds up. Besides the assessment fee, if you are accepted, there will be a weekly fee when you are attending group. It is a big commitment of your time, energy, and resources, so it's important to be sure that this is what you want to do. Sometimes women prefer the alternative of jail. Would you like to think about it more and get back to me?"
- "This is so unfair! All I did was throw a bottle at my boyfriend!" The therapist may respond: "Do you think that was OK, a good way to handle the situation?" or "Is this a relationship you care about and would like to see be better?" Pursuing somewhat more of a discussion in the initial phone contact can reveal the woman's attitude about her violence as well as possible motivators for her to participate in treatment.
- "What if I go to all this trouble and I don't get accepted? Do I get my money back?" The therapist can explain that the fee pays for the therapist's time, and can then ask her if she would like to know the criteria used to decide whether or not to accept her. (Rarely does anyone say no to this question!) The therapist can then explain that while the assessment interview covers a lot of territory (beginning to get to know her, her life experiences, what happened in the original incident that got her in trouble), the two most important things are:
  - Does she accept responsibility for her own behavior in the incident that led to her arrest? We do not expect her to take responsibility for her partner's behavior, but we do expect her to take responsibility for her own.
  - Does she want help?

The therapist can then suggest that the client give these questions some thought so she will be prepared for the assessment interview.

In these as well as all subsequent interactions, the therapist has the opportunity to model what the client will learn: staying calm when the other person is distressed, maintaining a clear sense of self and boundaries, and being nonreactive to another's anxiety. The therapist offers empathy as well as motivation to change.

The Initial Meeting

If the woman says she has the money for the assessment fee, then the therapist schedules her to come to the office within the next few days for a five-minute appointment. This is to pay the fee, schedule a return for the assessment interview, and receive the paperwork she must complete. Waiting longer to schedule this risks increasing the woman's anxiety or the possibility that she will not still have the money set aside for the assessment.

An additional important advantage of this brief meeting is that it allows the prospective client to see where the program's office is and to meet the therapist face-to-face. These earlier contacts provide the beginning of the therapeutic relationship and often help relieve some of the client's anxiety about the assessment interview. Often clients referred to a domestic violence program have never met with a therapist previously, have had negative experiences or negative preconceived expectations, or are feeling ashamed, defensive, and angry about being court-ordered to treatment.

The therapist gives the client a cover letter/receipt with the day and time to return for the assessment interview plus the packet of forms and releases (printed on program letterhead), emphasizing that she must be on time or early for this meeting because the whole time will be required. The assessment interview should be scheduled for the following week. The more quickly a woman makes it through this initial process and into group, the better.

Assessment Appointment Letter

Date: _____

To: _____

Address: _____

Dear _____:

This letter is to confirm your assessment appointment on _____ at _____. This letter also serves as your receipt that you have paid the assessment fee of $_____.

You must complete the enclosed forms and bring them with you to the meeting along with a pay stub from your most recent paycheck and/or your previous year income tax return.

Note: If you do not show for this assessment appointment, if you are late, or if you do not have the completed forms with you plus documentation about income, we will not do the assessment and you will not be refunded the assessment fee.

Your assessment will be held at my office at:

Entrance is:

Parking is available at:

When you arrive, please have a seat in the waiting room. The assessment interview will take one hour.

I look forward to meeting with you. If you have any questions, please feel free to contact me at my office (phone number) with times you can be reached.

Sincerely,

(Name of therapist)

Enc.

Intake Information

Name: _____ Date of birth: _____ ( ) Male ( ) Female

Address: (street, apt. number): _____

(city, state, zip code): _____

Telephone (home): _____   (cell): _____

(work): _____   (extension): _____

Occupation: _____   Employer: _____

Education: ( ) 1–12 years ( ) College (number of years): _____ Degree:_____

Other (trade school, professional training): _____

Marital status: ( ) Married, number of years: _____

( ) Separated ( ) Divorced   If so, when? _____

Number of previous marriages: _____

Children (names, ages, gender): _____

_____

Children live with: ( ) yourself

( ) someone else (relationship and name): _____

Spouse/Partner Information

Name: _____ Date of birth: _____ ( ) Male   ( ) Female

Telephone (home): _____ (cell): _____

(work): _____ (extension): _____

Occupation: _____   Employer: _____

Is this person the victim in your case?   ( ) yes   ( ) no

Name and phone number of victim, if different: _____

Program Rules

The purpose of this program is to help people stop their violent behavior. The therapist will teach about nonviolence, using role-play, handouts, video clips, and discussion to illustrate and facilitate a deeper understanding of concepts. Participants will have regular homework assignments.

Each group participant must adhere to the following rules:

- Attend 52 weeks of group meetings in not less than one year. Be on time. Lateness is disruptive and disrespectful to the rest of the group.
- If you arrive 10 minutes or more after group has begun, this will be considered an unexcused absence.
- Three tardies (late less than 10 minutes) equals one absence.
- Bring your binder (given to you at the assessment) to group each week. Any combination of three tardies or no binder equals one absence.
- No absences are allowed during the first 6 weeks.
- No more than four absences (or equivalents) are allowed. Absences are charged and must be made up in order to complete the program. If you must be absent, you must notify the therapist.
- All unexcused absences will be reported to probation. An absence is considered unexcused when the group member does not call the therapist *before* group and indicate *the reason* for the absence. Unexcused absences are not acceptable. If a participant has three unexcused absences or misses three meetings in a row, she will be immediately terminated from the program.
- Do not disclose what is said in group or reveal the names of those in attendance. Violating confidentiality will be grounds for immediate termination from the program.
- Pay for group meetings according to the agreement that you will sign at your assessment interview.
- Complete homework assignments. Homework turned in must never fall below 70% of the total assigned. If it does, this will count as the same as one absence.
- Special arrangements may be made with the therapist to take a vacation and miss not more than two group meetings. To qualify, the participant must be past the first six weeks, be current with fees and homework, clear the vacation dates with probation, and submit the request in writing to the therapist at least two weeks before leaving.
- The participant must complete 52 weeks of group in not more than 15 months from the first actual meeting to the last.
- Maintaining safety of all is a priority. Therefore, a participant must agree (1) to remove any guns and ammunition from home and vehicles while in this program, and (2) that volatile home situations take precedence over any other issues under discussion and must be reported during the next group meeting.
- The participant understands that the therapist is mandated by law to report any suspected child abuse or neglect, or any dependent elder abuse or neglect.

- The participant will not use any alcohol or drugs for a period of 12 hours before the start of group and 12 hours after the end of group. If the therapist assesses that there is a problem with substance abuse, the participant will be required to participate in a substance abuse treatment program.

The participant must agree to follow through with any referral recommended by the therapist. Referrals may include a psychological assessment, physical exam, neurological exam, or chemical dependency evaluation. Any such referral will be provided to the participant in writing, stating the type of evaluation, names and addresses of qualified professionals, and the reason for the referral. A copy of the referral will be provided to the probation department.

The participant must agree to work toward the goal of stopping domestic violence.

I have read and understand all of the program rules. I agree to abide by them.

_____   _____

Signature of participant   Date

Limits to Confidentiality

All information shared in group is confidential and shall not be shared outside of the group. No information will be released to anyone without your written consent. There are exceptions to your confidentiality protection as follows:

- A probation department representative may conduct an on-site review of the program. The purpose of the visit is to evaluate the program rather than the participation of any group member.
- The following information about you will be released to the court and/or probation department:
  a. Attendance and punctuality
  b. Participation in group
  c. Compliance with fee payments
  d. Additional acts of violence or threats of violence
- Sharing outside of group any personal information about other group members (including names) is strictly prohibited. This is a very serious matter and, if violated, will result in immediate termination from the program.
- If you continue to have contact with the victim or become involved in a new relationship, the therapist will want to have contact with that person. You will be asked to sign a release of information that authorizes the program to discuss your attendance, punctuality, participation in discussions, and completion of homework assignments. We will ask about your use of time-outs and ask about further acts of violence or threats of violence. The details of what you say in group will not be shared if they are not pertinent to the safety of your partner. You will not be told what your partner shares with the therapist.
- If the therapist determines that you are involved in neglecting, abusing, or otherwise endangering children, this will be reported to Child Protective Services and to probation. You will also be given the opportunity to report yourself.
- If you threaten to kill or hurt another person, according to existing laws, we are obligated to warn the potential victim as well as notify police.
- While in this program, if you are violent to your partner, we will report this to the police and to probation. We will encourage you to report your own offense. If we are subpoenaed by the court regarding the incident, confidentiality will be violated.

I have read and understand the above limits to confidentiality. I agree to the conditions as set forth.

_____   _____
Signature   Date

Waiver of Confidentiality to the Victim

This program holds all information received from participants in the strictest of confidence. Information will not be released without your permission.

It is our first priority to ensure safety of the victim; therefore, it is necessary that we contact him to monitor his safety.

The therapist will discuss only the following with the victim:

- Information about the program and its curriculum, including homework assignments and significant parts of the program that may affect the victim. The victim will be informed that violence in a relationship is a crime and that the police should be called and charges filed if violence occurs. If the therapist becomes aware of abuse, it is her responsibility to report the information to the police and probation.
- The victim will be told about your participation, whether you are taking the program seriously by participating in group discussions, completing homework assignments, and taking responsibility for behavior. Specifics of what you disclose in group will not be shared. Any direct threats you make against the victim will be shared with the victim. If the therapist thinks that the victim is in danger, he will be so notified.
- Information will be provided to the victim about community resources such as men's groups, shelters, child care, legal assistance, as well as whom to call in the event violence occurs.
- The victim will be told that just because you are participating in this program, no assurances are made that you may not become violent again.
- The victim will be asked to comment on whether he feels safe, and whether there has been any physical abuse or threats of abuse.
- You will not receive any information about what the victim has told program staff.

I, _____, hereby authorize this program to exchange the above confidential information with

_____

(Print victim's name)

_____

(Victim's phone number)

Consent for Treatment

I, _____, have read the program rules and limits of confidentiality.

I have agreed to waive confidentiality to the court and to the victim involved.

My questions have been answered concerning the program and I agree to abide by the conditions for acceptance.

By signing this consent for treatment, I am agreeing and/or acknowledging that I need to learn nonviolent and nonabusive ways of relating to others with whom I have intimate relationships.

My signature acknowledges that I understand all of the terms and conditions of this program.

_____   _____

Signature   Date

Assessment Interview

Ideally, by the time of the assessment interview, the client has already had a few interactions with the therapist.

This interview is critically important. It serves to:

- Further establish the therapeutic alliance—something that is especially helpful before the woman joins the group
- Obtain the client's perspective on what happened that led to her being referred to the program
- Obtain life history information about the client
- Determine if she needs other substance abuse or mental health treatment, and whether this should happen before entering the group or concurrently with group attendance
- Determine what type of relationship she has been in (i.e., one where she is primarily the victim, primarily the aggressor, or mutually abusive)
- Assess safety issues for her, her children, her partner
- Assess her motivation and suitability for treatment
- Offer hope that she can make her life, self, and relationships better

The following is a topical outline for the interview, with sample questions for each section. Because so much information is obtained, it is recommended that the therapist take copious notes during the interview. The notes then become a part of the client's chart and can be easily referenced over the course of the client's participation in the program.

The interview usually takes one hour but may last 1½ hours, especially if the woman has a significant history of trauma. First, review the paperwork packet she has returned, be sure that it is complete, and ask if she has any questions about what she has signed.

The therapist may then begin by saying:

> This interview is not only to decide if you are going to be accepted into our program, but also to begin to get to know you. I have a lot of questions I'm going to be asking you—not only about the incident that got you here, but also questions to begin to get to know you, your history, what has shaped you and led you to who you are today. This is a fairly structured interview in that I am going to follow this form that I have and write down everything you tell me. Because I have so much territory to cover, it actually works more efficiently if you bear with me and let me ask in the order I have my questions on the form. OK? I promise that if there is anything more that I haven't asked and that you think is essential for

me to know, you can tell me at the end of the interview. [But usually people feel like I've asked everything there is to know and more!]

Current Living Situation

- Whom do you live with (i.e., relationship, number of people)? How long? Whom did you live with before? How long?

You want to know if she's living with the domestic violence victim, with his children, her children, friends, or in a sober living environment (SLE). If this is a temporary living arrangement, you want to know when she plans to move, to what type of situation, and whether that new situation will be safe, provide stability, and support her in making her life better.

Children

- Ages and genders of children? Attending school? Where? How are they doing? Who takes care of the children? What is the custody/visitation arrangement? Is visitation supervised or not? Where is their father? What is their relationship like with him?

These questions help assess her view of her relationship with her own children. Children can be a strong, positive motivator for treatment. If a woman spent any time in jail, she probably was separated from her children. She may be especially worried about their welfare and want to protect them and to be a better mother.

Parents

- Are your parents still living? If one died, when? From what? How old were you? How did this affect you? Who comforted you?
- Are your parents still together? How long? Separations? Divorced? If so, what age were you?
- Why did they split up? How did you find out? How were you affected? Did either remarry? Who then raised you?

- Did any of your parents have problems with alcohol or drugs? Which parent? Did they get treatment? Maintain sobriety? How old were you then? How did this affect you?
- How did your parents argue with each other/resolve conflicts? Was there ever any domestic violence? Who was violent to whom? Where were you when this happened? How did this affect you? Were the police ever involved? Who called them? What was the outcome?
- What is your relationship like with your parents now?
- Do you want to have a marriage like your parents have? Why/why not?

Parents can be an important part of a woman's support system. They are also her earliest relationships. This information will start to tell you something about the woman's trauma history, her early attachment experiences, separations from parents, and how she learned to cope or not cope.

Siblings

- How many siblings? Where are you in the lineup? How did you get along with them growing up? How are your siblings doing in life now? Problems with alcohol or drugs? Domestic violence? Current relationships with siblings?

Siblings can also be an important part of a woman's support system. This history can tell you about the degree of dysfunction in the woman's family of origin, the roles each child played in the family, amount and type of trauma, attachment experiences, ability of family members to be resilient and recover.

Childhood

- Describe your childhood. What was it like?
- How did you get along with your parents and siblings?
- How were you punished when you were a child? For what kinds of things?
- Problems at school? Problems with the law?
- Were you molested as a child? By whom? Can you tell me about how this affected you?

These questions elicit information about early attachment experiences and the history and impact of trauma. The answers may also demonstrate the woman's ability to be self-disclosing, reflective, and psychologically minded.

Intimate Relationships History

- Previous marriages? Serious relationships? Living together?
- Why and how did those relationships end?
- Any domestic violence in those relationships? What type of violence? Who was violent to whom? Police involved? How did domestic violence affect the relationship?

Answers to these questions provide trauma history and help assess patterns in relationship experiences and the woman's ability to self-disclose and have insight about herself and how her history has affected her.

Current Domestic Violence Event (That Led Woman to Be Referred to Program)

- Tell me about what happened in the incident that led to you eventually being referred to this program. It is important that I understand the context of the situation, so please include when it first began and all of the details. (Ask chronologically: What happened? And then, what happened? Etc.)
- What got things started? What kept them going? Did you try to stop? Did your partner? What happened next?
- Why do you think this incident happened? How do you explain it to yourself?
- Did either of you have any injuries? What were they? Did they require medical attention?
- Where were the children? Have you talked to them about this? How did that go? How do you think they have been affected?
- Has this happened before? Police called? Who was violent to whom?
- Jail? How long? Restraining order? Modified or still in effect?

This information provides an understanding of the woman's perspective on what happened, her attitude about it—remorseful or defensive, justified. It enables evaluation of her minimization, denial, and blame; determines her role in the relationship—primarily the victim, primary aggressor, or mutually abusive; and assesses risk of lethality.

Mental Health History and Treatment

- Have you ever seen a therapist/counselor before? When? For how long? For what presenting problem? Was it helpful? If not, what didn't work/ went wrong?
- Have you ever felt like life was so overwhelming that you wished you could die?
- Have you ever tried to hurt or kill yourself? What did you do? What happened? How long ago was that?
- Psychiatric hospitalizations? When? What for?
- Are you currently taking *any* medications? Which? Dosage? How long? For what diagnosis? Is the medication helping you?

These questions assess risk of suicide and need for additional mental health treatment outside of group—either before starting group or concurrent with group participation. They assess the woman's attitude and expectations about therapy—positive and helpful or boring, unpleasant, intrusive, a waste of time.

Alcohol and Drug Use/Abuse/Treatment History

- When is the last time you had any alcohol? How much? Last time drunk?
- Age when you had your first drink? From then on, how often would you drink?
- When was the last time you used any drugs? Marijuana, speed/meth, cocaine, mushrooms, ecstasy, LSD, heroin, any others? Age when first used, how often, positive or negative experiences?
- Has alcohol or drug use ever caused other problems in your life (e.g., arguments with partners, trouble with the law, DUIs)?
- Have you ever attended AA or NA or other 12-step programs? Inpatient substance abuse treatment program? Which one? Did you complete it? What was discharge plan? Did you follow through?

- Do you think you are an addict? How long have you been clean and sober? Do you attend meetings? Which is your home meeting? Are you working with a sponsor? Which step?
- For addicts who are now clean and sober: How will I know or recognize that you have relapsed?

The greater a woman's history of trauma and insecure attachment experiences, the greater the likelihood she has also had problems with substance abuse. It is essential to know what her treatment needs might be in this area because the risk of relapse can be a great threat to her ability to benefit from her experience in the program and can jeopardize her ability to successfully complete the program.

Client's Goals for Treatment

- What would you like to gain from being in this program? What would you like help with?
- If you get what you want from this program, what would your relationship look like?
- How ready are you to do something to change (not ready, unsure, thinking about it, ready, very ready)?

These are the most important questions of the interview. Answers will give the therapist an indication of whether the woman thinks she has problems, sees that she has a role in the problems in her relationship, wants help, and takes responsibility for her part in what went wrong.

Additional Information?

- Is there anything I have neglected to ask you about that you believe is essential for me to know today?

Special Issues

- What if the woman arrives late for the assessment interview?

  Did she call ahead to say she was going to be late? Why is she late? If there has been a natural disaster (earthquake, tornado, flood) that interfered with her timely arrival, the therapist may decide to offer to reschedule the interview at no extra charge. In most cases, however, lateness to this appointment is an indication that the woman is not very motivated. If she is late to the assessment, especially when she has already been told that she must be on time, this lateness is likely to carry over to her arrival at group, and that is exceptionally disruptive to the group process. It is better to inform her that because she is late, she must forfeit the assessment fee, pay another, and reschedule.

- What if the woman brings her children to the interview?

Observing a woman interact with her children can reveal telling information about her. Sometimes women will say that their children can play quietly in a corner (this rarely happens for a whole hour) or that they are too young to understand what is being discussed (but even very young children sense a mother's emotional tone and may be distressed). So, it is not appropriate for children to be present at the interview. Both the woman and the therapist need to focus full attention on the content of the interview and not be distracted. If she brings her children, the woman should be told that the interview must be rescheduled for a time when her children are in school or with someone else who can watch them. If the woman is accepted into the program, she will have to arrange child care for them each week anyway.

- What if the woman forgot the paperwork or doesn't have it completed?

The paperwork contains releases and important agreements about her participation in the program. It is essential that she has read and signed them all, so she understands what will be expected of her. She forfeits the assessment fee and must pay again to reschedule.

- What if she appears to be under the influence of alcohol or drugs?

Sobriety is essential in order for a woman to benefit from this type of program. Sometimes, the therapist may be able to smell alcohol on the woman, and other times, the woman's speech may be slurred, incoherent, or the woman may lose her train of thought or even pass out during the interview. The therapist may simply tell the woman her concerns and that she wants to defer the decision about accepting or declining the woman until further discussion with the probation officer. This is the time to end the interview and recommend she contact her probation officer. Typically, a woman who shows up to an assessment interview under the influence of alcohol or drugs has a serious enough problem to warrant residential treatment. It may be a few months before she completes this, so she will need to start the assessment process over at that time (paying the fee, scheduling the interview). In the follow-up interview, it will be important to ask the woman about what she has been learning in rehab about herself and what relapse prevention plan is in place to support her in sobriety.

- What if she doesn't want to answer any questions? What if she is hostile or resistant?

Sometimes a woman may feel like she is being disloyal or betraying loved ones if she opens up to a near stranger about "family skeletons in the closet." The therapist may reassure her that while she does not need to know everything right now, if the woman is accepted into the program, she will be expected to, over time, open up in group about herself and consider how her history has affected her today. Most of the time, a reticent woman will be adequately reassured when the therapist explains the reasons certain information is asked and how it will be used. However, occasionally a woman is so overtly hostile that it is clear that she will not be able to participate constructively in group or may be disruptive to the group process. In this case, the woman should not be accepted into the program. The therapist can simply state that this is a therapeutic program and does not seem to be a good fit for what the woman wants. She is then referred back to her probation officer.

- Setting ground rules: What if the woman thinks her violence is acceptable, justified, entertaining, or humorous?

It is critical that the therapist remain self-aware and avoid giving what the client may interpret as mixed messages. She must retain a serious demeanor, no matter how cleverly or amusingly a woman may tell the story of her own violence. If the woman jokes about violence or makes excuses, the therapist can pause and say: "I want to be sure I am understanding you correctly. You seem to be making a joke about your behavior. Do you mean that you thought your violence was funny?" This is an opportunity to explore with the woman her underlying beliefs about women's and men's violence. Ultimately, the therapist must convey that violence is *never* an acceptable solution to relationship problems and, therefore, joking about violence is inappropriate.

How to Decide Whom to Accept

Several factors must be considered in deciding whom to accept into the program. A new client must be a good fit for the group as much as the group should be a good fit for her. As discussed earlier, she must accept responsibility for her own behavior in the incident that led to her arrest, and she must want help. This latter factor could be translated to mean that by the end of the assessment interview, she is at least at the contemplative stage of change, and hopefully even farther.

The therapist must also evaluate the woman's suitability to a group setting. Further questions to consider are these:

- Is she able to communicate in the language in which the group will be conducted?
- Is her current living situation stable enough to allow her regular attendance at group?
- Does she have transportation problems or work schedule conflicts?
- Will her child care needs allow for regular attendance at group?
- Does she have a drug or alcohol abuse problem that warrants more intensive treatment first?
- Does she have psychiatric problems that necessitate hospitalization, medication, or stabilization before joining a group? Is she suicidal or homicidal? Is she actively psychotic or delusional, so that the group experience may be too overwhelming and countertherapeutic for her?
- Is she able to interact appropriately enough to not be disruptive to the therapeutic experience for the other group members? Is she so hostile that it is clear she will be disruptive to the group?

At the conclusion of the assessment interview, the therapist has the following options:

- Accept the woman into the group
- Accept the woman contingent on her agreement to follow through with additional requirements (e.g., attending AA or NA meetings, getting a sponsor, and working the 12 steps)
- Defer acceptance until the woman has had further psychiatric assessment or her living situation is more stable
- Defer acceptance until the woman has completed residential substance abuse treatment, and then reassess

- Defer acceptance until discussion with the probation officer regarding any concerns about the woman's appropriateness to a group setting
- Deny acceptance and refer the woman back to probation

When a Client Is Accepted Into the Program

When the decision is made to accept a woman into the program, the therapist should tell her so and do the following:

- Determine her weekly fee for when she is attending group (using a sliding scale based on gross income and number of dependents).
- Have her sign two copies of the fee and payment policy: one for her chart and one for her records—to go in her program binder. (See Chapter 8 for form.)
- Give her a program binder. (Each group member is given a three-ring loose-leaf binder with copies of all program policies and rules, handouts, and so forth. The client is encouraged to keep in the binder all information pertinent to her participation in the program. As she receives returned copies of homework and progress reports, the binder is the best place to keep them.)
- Set a start date (preferably the next time the group meets).
- Point out two initial homework pages in the slot of the inner panel of the binder. These two pages are required and must be completed and turned in at the first group.
- Underscore the following points:
  - There *are* a lot of rules to follow in this program. I will not be going over all of them, because you have already signed a copy of them and have another copy in your binder. You will be held responsible for following them all.
  - Especially important, though, is to remember that you cannot miss any of the first six group meetings for any reason.
  - It is OK to be early or on time to group, but not OK to be late.
  - All fees must be paid in cash or money order (made out to the program).
  - No profanity or swearing is allowed in group. This is disrespectful and inflammatory language and counter to the program goal of communicating in a respectful way.
  - No alcohol or drug use 24 hours before group, or after group. If I suspect that you are under the influence, you will be asked to leave and that group meeting will count as an absence.
- Ask if she has any questions. Often, the client will ask what to expect at the first group meeting. The therapist may describe how many women are in the group and that they all sit in a big circle with the therapist. At the first meeting, the other group members will each introduce themselves to the new member, who will then be asked to tell her story to the

group as well as share her initial homework. If the group room is not in use, the therapist may show it to her.

- Ensure that the woman knows where to arrive for group.
- Emphasize the expectation that if, for any reason, she is unable to attend group, even if it means she will be terminated from the program, she should call the therapist to let her know that she is OK. The therapist might say: "Whenever someone doesn't show up for group, I worry about her because not being here usually means bad news—the woman is in jail, in a car accident in the ditch, unconscious at the hospital, in trouble somehow. So, I worry. Even if you forget to come to group and remember it in the middle of the night, I want you to call and leave me a message about what happened so I know you are OK. Even if this means you will be terminated from group (e.g., because of absence in the first six meetings), I will be more likely to try to work out something, like allowing you to restart the program. OK?"

After concluding the assessment interview, the therapist should fax a memo to probation or the referring judge indicating the outcome of the interview.

Memorandum: Proof of Enrollment

Date: _____

To: _____

    (Name of P.O. or judge)

From: _____ @ _____

    (Name of therapist and name of program)

_____ was referred to our domestic violence

treatment program by probation/court on _____.

( ) The client made an assessment appointment but failed to appear.

( ) The client had an assessment interview on _____ with the following results:

( ) Accepted into program, beginning group on _____.

( ) Not accepted into the program for the following reasons:

_____

_____

( ) Acceptance deferred until following issue(s) is addressed/resolved:

_____

_____

_____

_____ @ _____

    (Therapist's signature and phone number)

When a Client Is Not Accepted Into the Program

If, by the end of the assessment interview, the woman is still at the pre-contemplative stage, it is important for the therapist to remember that lecturing or warning is countertherapeutic and rarely elicits positive results. This program is based on the concept of client self-determination—the belief that every human being has a right to make her own decisions about her life. Different choices have different consequences, but no one can be forced to change. The therapist's role is to offer help and direction when the client is ready and *chooses* to change.

If a client decides not to begin the program, or the therapist decides to defer or deny acceptance into the program, the therapist should immediately call the probation officer to discuss reasons and recommendations for alternative treatment. This phone call should be followed by a faxed memo with the same information.

Contact With the Partner/Victim

Information provided by the woman's partner (the victim) is also important for assessing her progress. For women court-ordered to treatment, this contact is likely to be defined and mandated by state domestic violence laws.

The client signs a waiver of confidentiality to the victim as part of the paperwork she brings to her assessment interview. After she has been accepted into the program, the therapist contacts the client's partner by phone.

The focus of contact should be to explain the program and aspects that may affect him (e.g., time-outs), ascertain if he feels safe, urge him to take violence seriously and protect himself appropriately (e.g., calling police, seeking legal action such as restraining orders), and encourage him to seek his own counseling. The therapist provides him with information about community resources for domestic violence victims. He is also given contact information for the program therapist should he later have further questions or want to share concerns about his partner's behavior.

Male victims of domestic violence may be reluctant or ambivalent about speaking with their female partner's therapist. They cannot be required to participate in their own counseling, and their contact with the program should be based on their willingness to speak. It is important to convey to them that a wife or girlfriend's participation in the program does not guarantee that she will not be violent again.

My own experience is that male partners generally tend to be less willing to speak to a program therapist than their female counterparts. Also, some of the men have enrolled in or completed their own court-ordered domestic violence treatment programs before their wives or girlfriends have been arrested. These situations illustrate in a compelling way how domestic violence is a relationship or family issue that warrants interventions that address the whole family.

What if the partner doesn't want to talk to the therapist and hangs up on her?

Answer: He has a right to not participate in any discussion about himself and his wife or girlfriend. The therapist must respect this.

What if he complains to the therapist that the legal system has ruined their family because now *he* has to pay for his wife to go to this program and they were handling their problems just fine by themselves?

Answer: The therapist can respond sympathetically. She acknowledges that this experience can create hardships for families, and she hopes that his wife will benefit from the program—ultimately benefitting their relationship and their family.

What if he tells the therapist that his alcoholic girlfriend is still drinking (in violation of the terms of her probation and requirements of the program)?

Answer: Partners may have complex and varied motives for making a report of substance abuse. A partner may be telling the truth and be genuinely worried, or he may be lying and wanting to get his wife/girlfriend in trouble. He may want to test the therapist to see how she will respond, or he may want to see if what he tells the therapist gets back to his wife/girlfriend.

The therapist must be cautious in responding so that she does not unwittingly place herself in the middle of the couple's drama. She expresses concern and yet *focuses on him and his plans* for his own and his children's safety. AlAnon can be a valuable resource for him and she urges him to attend.

She owes him no explanation of what she will do with his information. In addition, she does not tell his wife/girlfriend that they have spoken or what he said.

From information obtained in the assessment interview, the therapist should know the woman's risk of ongoing substance abuse and should periodically check with her about her recovery (i.e., attending AA or NA meetings, working with a sponsor, etc.). How does the woman think her recovery is going? What aspects are difficult for her? What would she like help with?

Concerns about possible ongoing substance abuse or relapse should also be addressed with the probation officer.

What if he says that his wife/girlfriend is still being violent?

Answer: The therapist expresses concern for his safety and that of the children. She asks what happened and urges him to contact police to make a report and speak to the woman's probation officer. Family safety is the highest concern. The therapist does not ask the woman to respond to her partner's report; in fact, she does not indicate that the partner even spoke to her, let alone what he said. She remains alert to what the woman is sharing in group and recognizes that her version of an event may be different from her partner's. The partner's report of continued violence should be shared and discussed with the probation officer to formulate an appropriate therapeutic intervention.

What if he wants to know what his wife/girlfriend says about him in group?

Answer: The therapist reminds him that all specific information shared in group is confidential. Is there a certain concern that he has? Would he like to share this with the therapist? This can be an opportunity to redirect the partner to seeking his own support and counseling.

What if he shows up at group and demands to speak to his wife/girlfriend?

Answer: This situation poses a potential risk to safety and certainly to anonymity of group members. It is absolutely inappropriate and disrespectful, no matter how justified the partner thinks he is. The therapist must politely and firmly guide the partner out of the group room and building before listening to his concerns. Our group room also has a landline telephone for emergency phone calls.

8

Record Keeping and Administrative Forms

Documenting and keeping track of paperwork can be overwhelming when doing a group like this. This chapter provides all of the forms necessary plus a system for efficiently managing paperwork. The purpose of this is to streamline record keeping so more attention and energy can be available for doing the therapy. All forms are presented in the order in which they are used.

Various documents or forms are kept in four places for each client:

1. Client's chart
2. Client's folder
3. Client's binder
4. Sign-in notebook

The **client's chart** contains five sections:

1. Correspondence
2. Program forms (signed by client)
3. Assessment interview notes and treatment plan
4. Homework
5. Case notes and progress reports

The chart is a manila folder with metal tabs on the top left and right sides and papers punched with two holes at the top to fit tabs. Each section is divided by a color-coded tab. The "Contents of Chart" form is glued on the outside cover.

On the left side (from bottom up when folder is open) are correspondence and program forms, topped with an intake information page. On the right side (from bottom up when folder is open) are assessment and treatment plan, homework, and case notes. As progress reports are written, they are inserted on top of the right side, so they are easily found when the folder is opened.

This chart is filed in a locked cabinet in a secure area of the office, accessible only to program staff.

The following is printed on a half-sheet of 8½ × 11 paper and glued to the outside of the client's chart. As each item is added to the chart, the therapist checks it off. This provides a handy snapshot of the chart.

Contents of Chart

Date of first group: _____ Date of Last group: _____

( ) Probation department referral
( ) Pre-sentence report from probation
( ) Proof of enrollment
( ) Treatment plan
( ) Victim contacts

Dates: _____   _____   _____
     Whereabouts unknown ( )
( ) Case notes
( ) Progress reports

Dates: _____   _____

              _____   _____

              _____   _____

( ) Final evaluation   Date: _____

Treatment Plan

Date: _____

Client: _____ Therapist: _____

Client's statement (from assessment interview—what she said she wants help with):
Treatment plan objectives —Client will:
1.   Stop violent behavior.
Comments:

2.   Accept responsibility for violent behavior—without minimization, denial, or blame.
Comments:

3.   Demonstrate emotional self-awareness and insight, the ability to regulate her own emotions through healthy self-talk, and the ability to choose nonviolence.
Comments:

4.   Demonstrate understanding of domestic violence, forms of abuse in relationships, and the effects on families, relationships, victims, and children.
Comments:

5.   Improve communication skills and how to partner in a relationship based on equality. Demonstrate respectful problem-solving skills, time-outs, and respectful language and behavior.
Comments:

6.   Continue substance abuse recovery program with reports of attendance as appropriate.
Comments:

7.   Take responsibility for her own safety and welfare, and that of her children.
Comments:

Progress Report

Faxed to P.O. _____ on _____

_____ _____ _____
Participant's name   Date of birth   Date of this report

_____ _____ _____
Date of assessment   Date started group   Group day/time

Current status: Currently enrolled _____ Terminated date _____

Restart date _____ Suspension date _____ Date reinstated _____

Attendance: Total attended: ____ Total tardies: ____ Total "no binder": ____
Total absences: ____ Excused: ____ Unexcused: ____ Absences remaining: __

Participation: (circle all that apply) Denial Disruptive Resistant Minimizes

Blames   Inconsistent   Inattentive   Cooperative   Respectful

Self-discloses   Asks for advice   Demonstrates empathy   Attentive/engaged

Positive influence in group   Demonstrates insight about own behavior

Homework:
Amount assigned _____ Amount completed _____ Homework % _____
Doesn't understand Minimal Fair Trying to understand Good Exceptional

Progress: (circle all that apply)   No evidence of progress   Recent violence
Unsafe situation Minimal progress Understands time-outs Takes time-outs
Uses respectful language and behavior
Demonstrates: Respectful   Problem-solving skills   Self-awareness
Self-responsibility

Fees: Amount _____ Balance owed _____ Number of warnings _____
Substance abuse treatment required: Yes ____ No ____ Recommended ____

Program _____

Comments: _____

_____

_____ _____ _____
Therapist name (print)   Therapist's signature   Date

The **client's folder** contains a two-sided "Attendance Log" form where the therapist records after each group meeting: attendance, tardies, homework, fees paid. Clients do not write on this.

Taped inside the folder is an envelope where the client places fee payment each week.

Before group, the folders for all group members are placed on a table in the group room for the women to place fees and homework. After group, the therapist gathers them and records information.

The folders then are stored in the locked, secure cabinet with the charts.

Attendance Log

Name: _____ **Weekly fee:** _____ **P.O.:** _____

AA or NA meetings required? _____ **Number per week:** _____

HOMEWORK

Date	Attendance	Due	In	%	Amount Due	Payment	Balance
1.							
2.							
3.							
4.							
5.							
6.							
7.							
8.							
9.							
10.							
11.							
12.							
13.							
14.							
15.							
16.							
17.							
18.							
19.							
20.							
21.							
22.							
23.							
24.							
25.							
26.							

Name: _____ **Weekly fee:** _____ **P.O.:** _____

HOMEWORK

Date	Attendance	Due	In	%	Amount Due	Payment	Balance
27.							
28.							
29.							
30.							
31.							
32.							
33.							
34.							
35.							
36.							
37.							
38.							
39.							
40.							
41.							
42.							
43.							
44.							
45.							
46.							
47.							
48.							
49.							
50.							
51.							
52.							

Extra Group Meetings to Make Up for Absences

The **client's binder** is given to the client at the end of the assessment interview when she is accepted into the program. It is a one-inch three-ringed binder with a clear pocket on the front and pockets on either side inside.

In the outside pocket, place a cover page with the name of the program, name and phone number of the group therapist, and client's name.

Women often personalize their binders by inserting photos of children and loved ones. Initial homework is placed in the left inside pocket. Woman are strongly encouraged to keep in this binder all paperwork related to the program (e.g., copies of progress reports, correspondence from probation, homework, AA/NA meeting attendance forms).

Following the welcome letter, the rest of the binder is divided into six sections, as follows. (The forms for the welcome letter, fees and payment policy, group rules, and requirements for completion of the program follow this list. Additional forms included in the binder are included in Chapter 10 with discussion of their use in group.)

Section 1: Policies and rules
- Fees and payment policy
- Program rules
- Limits to confidentiality
- Waiver of confidentiality to victim
- Group rules
- Requirements for completion of program

Section 2: Domestic violence
- Ten truths
- Domestic violence: The expanded definition
- Responsibility and empowerment
- Comparing relationships: Equality versus power and control
- Am I safe?
- Physical cues: The brain and the anger response
- Time-outs
- Tranquility breathing

Section 3: Homework
- How to do journal homework
- Example of journal homework
- Emotions inventory
- Self-talk: Inflammatory versus calming
- "Making motion pictures"
- Examples of calming self-talk

Section 4: Relationship issues
- Jealousy
- A meaningful apology
- Forgiveness
- Empathy
- Boundaries
- Sex and intimacy
- Coping with criticism
- Understanding assertiveness
- Constructive conflict and problem solving
- Cycle of violence

Section 5: Family of origin
- Family of origin
- Coherent narrative
- Attunement and attachment
- Four attachment styles
- Effects of domestic violence on children
- Parenting nonviolently: Teaching our children
- Co-parenting with an ex-partner

Section 6: Inspiration
- Letting go
- Serenity prayer

Welcome Letter

Dear _____,

Welcome!

This binder is yours to keep. Bring it to group each week and use the information enclosed to help you with homework and the principles that this program stands for. The binder information is divided into six sections: policies and rules, domestic violence, how to do anger journals, relationship skills, family of origin, and inspiration.

Your first group meeting is _____ at _____.

Your weekly fee is $_____. This must be paid each week by cash or money order made out to this program.

For your first group meeting, be sure you complete the homework (located in the inside left pocket of this binder).

If you ever need to reach me, call me at _____. I will either answer the phone or return your message as soon as possible.

I look forward to working together with you!

(Therapist signature)

Two copies are signed by client and therapist: one for the chart and one for the client's binder.

Fees and Payment Policy

The fee for the assessment interview is $_____ for all applicants to this program. This fee is nonrefundable, whether or not you are accepted into this program.

At the end of the assessment interview, if you are accepted into the program, your therapist will establish your weekly fee. You will be expected to pay the amount agreed upon each week until you have completed the program. You owe the weekly fee whether or not you attend group.

If you do not pay for a two-week period, a pretermination letter will be sent to you with a copy to your probation officer.

If you do not pay the fees due by the next group meeting, you will be suspended from the program for three weeks and your probation officer will be notified. You will not be charged for the three-week suspension.

If you *do not* pay the fees due by the three-week deadline, you will be terminated from the program. If you *do* pay the fees by the deadline, and you fall behind again, you will be terminated from the program and not allowed to return to restart the program until all past due fees are paid in full.

Weekly fees are determined according to a sliding scale, based on gross income and number of dependents. Verification of income is required in order to qualify for reduced fees.

Your fees must be paid in cash or money order made out to this program. Personal checks are not accepted.

Participants in the program are responsible for outstanding fees, even after they are no longer in the program.

_____
Weekly fee

_____   _____
Group participant's signature   Date

_____   _____
Therapist's signature   Date

Initial Homework

(2 pages)

Name _____ Date _____

Answer the following and bring with you to your first group meeting. Be prepared to share this information with the rest of the group.

1. **Personal goals**
   List three personal goals you want to work on during this next year, not related to this program (e.g., related to job, employment, education, self-sufficiency).

   (1)

   (2)

   (3)

2. **Goals for this program**
   List three goals you have for while you are in this program (e.g., problems you want help with—What do you want to improve about yourself? What do you want to learn?).

   (1)

   (2)

   (3)

3. **Things I can do to reach my goals**
   For each of the above goals (related to this program), write three ideas you have for specific things you can do that will help you begin to achieve those goals.

   (1)

   (2)

   (3)

Initial Homework

(continued)

Name _____   Date _____

When you start to feel angry, what physical sensations do you start to feel in your body (e.g., hotness, fast heartbeat, knot in stomach, tense muscles, headache, sweaty palms, etc.)?

Where do the physical feelings begin and where do they travel as you get more angry?

What is a physical signal that you experience right before you lose it with your anger?

What kinds of situations or experiences push your buttons or really get under your skin? What is especially upsetting to you that is like a trigger for your anger? (Discuss.)

Requirements for Completion of Program

To our clients:

The following information is provided to help you understand our expectations of you and how we will determine that you have completed the objective of our program.

While some may be tempted to think of completion of the program as like a graduation, we instead view it as the beginning of a journey—a journey on the path of equality and nonviolence. We expect that through participation in this program, you will continue to change even after you are no longer attending group meetings: continuing to examine your behavior, underlying beliefs, and intentions; taking responsibility for the choices you make; being accountable for yourself; and holding others accountable for themselves. It is the responsibility of all of us to stop violence.

Given this, successful completion of this program will be determined when you:

1. Have completed a minimum of 52 group meetings in no less than one year
2. Have been violence-free for a minimum of 6 months
3. Have cooperated and participated in the program (i.e., group discussions, role-plays, homework assignments, etc.)
4. Have demonstrated an understanding and use of positive, nonviolent conflict resolution skills
5. Do not blame, degrade, or do anything that dehumanizes others or places their safety at risk
6. Have demonstrated acceptance of responsibility for your own behavior

In addition to these requirements, you must also be up-to-date with payment of your group fees.

Before each group meeting, a spiral notebook is left alongside the folders. This is the **sign-in notebook** and provides verification of attendance and informs the therapist of each woman's next court review date or next meeting with her probation officer.

Progress reports to probation are written two weeks before either of these events, so that the woman may have her own copy well beforehand.

Each woman is to sign in before group (see sample sign-in page). After group, this notebook is stored with the charts and folders.

When completing the chart for the upcoming group, the therapist lists the names of women who are scheduled to be at group.

Sign-In

Women's Group

Date: _____

Print Name	Next Court Date	Signature
1.		
2.		
3.		
4.		
5.		
6.		
7.		
8.		
9.		
10		
11.		
12.		

Additional forms are provided here for when a client is not in compliance with program requirements. These circumstances are spelled out in the program rules, which the client signs before the assessment interview.

The forms are "Pretermination Warning Letter" and "Termination Letter." In both cases, the therapist completes the form, faxes a copy to the probation officer or judge, sends a copy to the client, and keeps the original in the client's chart.

Pretermination Warning Letter

Date: _____

Participant name: _____

Address: _____

Our records indicate you are out of compliance with the agreement(s) you made as a condition for your participation in this program. You are not in compliance in the following area(s):

( ) Unexcused absences
Comments:

( ) Lack of fee payment
Comments:

( ) Homework assignments not turned in
Comments:

( ) Other
Comments:

In order to remain enrolled in this program, you must contact your group therapist at _____ and bring the above item(s) into compliance by your next group meeting on _____. If you do not, you will be terminated from this program. If it is your decision to withdraw, please notify us. A copy of this letter is also being sent to your probation officer.

Respectfully,

(Therapist signature)

Termination Letter

Date: _____

Participant name: _____

Address: _____

Our records indicate you are out of compliance with the agreement(s) you made as a condition for your participation in this program. You are not in compliance in the following area(s):

( ) Unexcused absences
Comments:

( ) Lack of fee payment
Comments:

( ) Homework assignments not turned in
Comments:

( ) Other
Comments:

You have not taken the necessary action to bring yourself into compliance with program requirements. Therefore, you are hereby terminated from this program. A copy of this letter is being sent to your probation officer. You must contact him/her regarding your status with the court. If you have further questions, you may contact us at _____.

Respectfully,

(Therapist signature)

When the therapist determines that a client needs substance abuse treatment and that outpatient treatment will be adequate, she may require that the client attend a certain number of AA or NA (or other 12-step) meetings per week.

Sometimes probation officers or a judge may require 12-step meeting attendance but only require that a client obtain a signature from the secretary of the meeting. I have found it more therapeutic, instead, to expect a client to write about each meeting she attended and what she got out of the meeting.

The following page is a form for the woman to complete and turn in each week at group.

12-Step Meeting Response Form

Name _____ Date of next group meeting _____

Type of 12-step meeting I attended this week (i.e. AA, NA, SLAA, etc.): _____

Day, time, and place of 12-step meeting: _____

One idea I heard at this meeting and want to remind myself of: _____

_____

12-Step Meeting Response Form

Name _____ Date of next group meeting _____

Type of 12-step meeting I attended this week (i.e. AA, NA, SLAA, etc.): _____

Day, time, and place of 12-step meeting: _____

One idea I heard at this meeting and want to remind myself of: _____

_____

12-Step Meeting Response Form

Name _____ Date of next group meeting _____

Type of 12-step meeting I attended this week (i.e. AA, NA, SLAA, etc.): _____

Day, time, and place of 12-step meeting: _____

One idea I heard at this meeting and want to remind myself of: _____

_____

When a woman has four group meetings remaining for completion of meeting requirements, she is given her final homework (three pages). This is to be completed over the next few weeks and turned in at her next-to-last group meeting.

A copy of this final homework is attached to the final evaluation and given to the woman at her last group meeting.

The final evaluation is faxed to probation and the original is kept in the client's chart.

Final Homework: For Completion of Program

(three pages)

Describe in detail the incident that led to your arrest and referral to this program.

Describe in detail how you would deal differently with the same circumstances should they occur today. Be specific.

Final Homework: For Completion of Program

What have you learned about yourself and how have you changed as a result of participating in this program? Be specific.

Give five examples from the last month of how you have used the new relationship and coping skills you have been learning (i.e., examples in which you dealt differently with a situation than you would have in the past).

Final Homework: For Completion of Program

What is it going to be like not attending group anymore?

Review the personal and program goals you set for yourself when you first started here. Which have you accomplished and which do you want to continue to work toward?

What commitment do you make to continue the changes and personal growth you have been working on in this program?

What will you recognize as warning signs that you need to seek help again? (Be specific.) What actions will you then take?

Final Evaluation

Faxed to P.O. _____ on _____

_____ _____ _____
Participant's name   Date started group   Date of final group

Total attended: _____ Total absences: _____ ( ) All fees are paid in full

According to available information, _____ has been free of
physical violence for a minimum of six months. In addition:

( ) She has been cooperative in her participation and compliant with program requirements and group rules.
Comments:

( ) She has demonstrated motivation to change and a commitment to the principles of
nonviolence in relationships.
Comments:

( ) She takes responsibility for her behavior and does so without minimization, denial, or
blame. She is able to recognize her own part in conflicts and problems.
Comments:

( ) She demonstrates understanding of domestic violence, forms of abuse in relationships,
and the effects on families, relationships, victims, and children. She demonstrates empathy and respect for self and others.
Comments:

( ) She has demonstrated the ability to share power and control in relationships. She uses
time-outs, respectful problem-solving skills, language, and behavior.
Comments:

( ) She demonstrates emotional self-awareness and insight, the ability to regulate her own
emotions through healthy self-talk, and the ability to choose nonviolence.
Comments:

( ) She takes responsibility for her own safety and welfare, and that of her children.
Comments:

Additional concerns and recommendations: _____

_____

_____

_____ _____
Therapist's signature   Date

Suggested Information for Charts or Posters Displayed in Group Room

Check-in

1. Are you experiencing a crisis that you would like help with?
2. Have you experienced violence this last week (that you committed, participated in, witnessed, or experienced)?
3. Do you have an issue or situation about which you would like advice?
4. What progress are you making in accomplishing the goals you set for yourself when you began this program?

Wrap-up

1. What do you think about how group went today? What did you like? What would have made the group more helpful to you personally?
2. If you did not get what you needed, what would have been helpful for you?
3. What did you hear or learn in group today that you intend to apply in your own life?
4. What commitment do you make to the group about following through on advice you were given today?

Additional posters might include the ten truths, five guarantees, serenity prayer, cycle of violence, group rules, and the phrase "Acknowledge feelings, choose behavior."

9

Facilitating the Group
Getting Started

Education and the Group Therapy Model

Group therapy offers women a powerful experience to help them better understand themselves and others. It is infinitely more effective than if these same women were in individual treatment for the same issues. Hearing the same message from a room full of women she has come to respect—because they care about her and have also been in her shoes—is considerably more motivating than hearing the same message from a single therapist.

The group becomes a smaller representation of the culture at large, modeling to each woman pro-social behaviors. The group offers a reparative experience, a safe place; to experience belonging to a community in the face of isolation and shame; to explore intense and overwhelming feelings; to be cared for and at the same time have faulty beliefs challenged; to be fully present for a person who is speaking and at the same time manage her own anxiety; experience attunement, empathy, compassion, and, respect; and in turn, to demonstrate these qualities to others.

In many ways, therapy is more art than science. While specific skills are taught, the greatest education is experiential within the context of the group. The therapist as facilitator is responsible for setting the tone for this experience, providing structure and direction and modeling appropriate behavior. Women will remember the deeper experience of the group—feeling safe, accepted, valued, respected, and competent—longer than the specific skills they are taught. Process will always be more significant than content.

These responsibilities may seem daunting, but the therapist can do some specific things to facilitate this. While it may initially seem awkward, women should raise their hands to speak and wait to be called on. Similar to directing an orchestra, the therapist uses pacing and leading to guide how deeply issues are explored and discussed, which women are encouraged to participate more, and which are encouraged to listen more.

Because many abusive women also have borderline personality disorder, it is critically important that the therapist be reliable and consistent from week to week (be on time, follow structure and format, be predictable). The therapist must remain clearly in charge and feel comfortable exercising her authority to keep the group safe and focused on the purpose of the group.

Good therapy is also good education. These groups are intentionally designed to be open-ended, meaning that each group has women who are newer, who are in the middle of the program, and who are close to completion. Because we learn best what we in turn teach to someone else, this allows more senior members to pass on their knowledge and wisdom to newer members.

If discussions are relevant to the women's lives, they will pay closer attention and want to learn. When they connect personally with the content that is presented, when it has meaning for them, they will be engaged and more willing to examine themselves and want to change.

Basic Format and Structure of Group Meetings

Because the women's beginnings and completions of the program are staggered throughout the ongoing group, these events are woven with ongoing issues already being addressed in group meetings.

Structure of Group Meeting

Chairs are set evenly spaced in a circle around the room. On the walls are posters of the ten truths, five guarantees, serenity prayer, cycle of violence, group rules, and check-in and wrap-up guidelines. In the center is a table holding the sign-in notebook, an individual folder for each woman, pens and Post-it notepads (should a woman want to leave a note for the therapist), Kleenex, and blank journal homework forms.

Before a group starts, each woman adds her signature to the sign-in notebook page for that date and notes the date of her next court review. She also places her fees, homework, and, if required, AA/NA meeting response forms inside her personal folder. If a progress report has been written for an upcoming court review, her copy will be in her folder for her to read and take. Women are urged to put these reports in their program binders and take them to court—in case the copy sent to probation or the judge has been mislaid.

Each group meeting lasts for two hours and has a five-minute break halfway through.

Group starts on time, and everyone is expected to be in her seat and ready. The therapist may make a few brief announcements, for example, announce journal homework is due, welcome a new member, acknowledge a member who is close to completing the program, announce holiday schedule if group is not meeting or therapist will be on vacation, explain a member's absence and report on her safety. The therapist may also use this time to return copies of homework (on which she has made comments).

Note: Group members should be given written notice of holiday or therapist vacation dates at least a month in advance along with information about emergency contact in the therapist's absence.

The therapist then formulates the plan for the meeting by triage. Precedence is given to any member who is currently experiencing a crisis and needs support and direction. Safety is always the priority, and group members are encouraged and expected to advocate for themselves with the therapist and group by asking for group time to discuss their concerns. Other group members may sometimes speak up for a more timid one, telling the therapist that they know a particular member has something she needs to be talking about in group.

When the plan for the meeting is determined, as a warm-up the therapist may ask everyone to open her binder and turn to a particular page, which is then read and discussed. Then the group moves to group time: check-in, discussion, role-plays of members' examples of situations.

The therapist has several options for each group meeting:

- Headline check-in. Each woman briefly gives a headline (one sentence) summary of a problem she is dealing with in life; something she needs help with; a success she wants to share; a crisis she has experienced; a report of any violence she has perpetrated, experienced, or witnessed, or a new realization about herself and her relationships. This brief check-in allows the therapist to triage—to organize group time so that the most urgent problems are addressed in adequate depth and still discover at least a little about how each woman is doing in life.

- Asking who needs group time. If a woman has called the therapist between group meetings, the therapist should have not only helped her with immediate support, crisis intervention, and problem solving, but also asked her to tell the rest of the group at the next meeting. If a woman has had police contact, Child Protective Services contact, or violence in the last week, this calls for mandatory check-in.
- Asking group members to nominate women to share who have not opened up in group. Ask the nominators to frame their questions to the nonparticipating members.
- Reviewing and discussing of handout material in the program binder. Depending on the topic, this may be brief, taking only 10 to 15 minutes, or it may take up most of the group time (as when family of origin is shared).
- Asking each woman to share an entry from her anger journal and facilitate a discussion of each.
- Posing a question to the group and facilitate a discussion.

Because women tend to be quite verbal, a therapist may find that rather than trying to elicit discussion, everyone wants to talk at the same time, and there is never enough time for the topics women bring as well as topics that the therapist wants to address. In this case, it is important to remember that there are many routes to learning the same information; discussing educational material through the context of the women's real-life experiences will always be the most effective. Therefore, women's issues should always be given precedence over simply reading over and discussing handouts in the program binder. This does necessitate the therapist's being quick on her feet, creative, and able to readily improvise.

About halfway through the group meeting and at a good stopping point in the discussion, the therapist announces break time. This five minutes allows for women to visit the bathroom, get water or coffee, take a quick walk outside, or have a cigarette (if local ordinances and program policy allow for smoking outside of the building). Although this might seem like a distraction from the therapeutic process, women typically talk together during this time and connect in valuable ways that actually enhance the formal group experience. In a smaller group and away from earshot of the therapist, women may open up more to seasoned group members, who then can respond with helpful advice and encouragement to bring the issue to group.

This break also allows time for the therapist to speak individually to a group member about private issues that are not appropriate for the rest of the group (e.g., falling behind in fees or homework) or issues that the therapist may prefer to address first individually rather than in the group forum (e.g., a woman's attitude, body language, suspicions of substance abuse). In turn, it is also a time for women to speak individually with the therapist about their own concerns that are not appropriate to the group as a whole (e.g., therapist's comments on progress reports to the judge, requests to modify fees).

For the second half of group, the therapist may continue the discussion of the previous topic or move on to addressing other members' concerns.

About 15 minutes before the scheduled end of group, the therapist begins wrap-up. Going around the circle, each woman is asked to reflect on the group meeting today, sharing how she thinks group went and why, and something that she learned for herself or is going to apply in her life. Wrap-up comments give valuable feedback to the therapist about how members experienced a group, and whether they heard what the therapist had hoped for.

Sometimes during wrap-up, a woman may be tempted to use this time to give further advice to other group members or to comment on their progress (or lack thereof). This should be strongly discouraged. Wrap-up is a time for each woman to focus on herself, to contemplate her own internal life, who she wants to be and how she wants to change.

An Important Note About Homework

Homework is mandatory, not optional. Initial homework focuses a woman's attention on awareness of herself and her physical cues of anger and triggers, as well as her personal goals and program goals. This is to be turned in as well as shared in her first group meeting.

Thereafter, journal homework is to be completed one entry per week and turned in every four weeks (as indicated in each woman's log in her folder and announced in group). Regular practice of this exercise helps a woman improve her self-awareness and ability to regulate her emotions, and empowers her to better control her own behavior.

The final homework is required in order to complete the program. It is given out one month before the last group meeting and is due at least one week before the last group meeting. In this homework, the woman is asked to reflect on what she originally did to bring her to the program, what she has learned, and how she would respond differently given the same circumstances. This homework is shared at her last group meeting and is added to her final evaluation upon completing the program.

When First Establishing a New Group

While the ideal size for this type of group is 10 to 12, a new group can be started with three or four women, adding new members as they are accepted into the program.

At the beginning of the first meeting, the therapist welcomes the women who are starting this new group and provides initial orientation to the format for the group (two hours, check-in, five-minute break halfway through, wrap-up at end of group) and group rules and expectations.

She may have the women turn to the binder page entitled "Domestic Violence: The Expanded Definition," then have the women read and discuss their reactions: Do you agree? Do you see yourself here? Your partner? What are the effects of the different types of abuse? Why do you think we consider these to be examples of domestic violence? What is most important here is to encourage women to feel safe in expressing their thoughts and opinions, even if they disagree with the therapist. This is also an opportunity for them to be more reflective about *what* they believe and *why*.

The therapist encourages the women, if they have not already done so, to become familiar with the information in their binders and notes that in the next few group meetings they will be discussing many topics contained in binder handouts.

She then explains that because this is the very first group, it is important for the group members to begin to get to know each other. Each woman is asked to introduce herself along with an expanded description of the incident that led to her arrest. The therapist may first explain that the purpose of this is to begin to get to know each other, and for each woman to take responsibility for her own behavior. "We recognize that each person's situation is invariably complicated, with many factors that led up to or contributed to the eventual violence. Some of you may have been abused by your partner and may feel unfairly accused, some of you may have a history of mutual violence with your partner, and for some of you, this may be the first time you were ever violent. We do not expect you to take responsibility for your partner's or anyone else's bad behavior, but we do expect you to take responsibility for your own. When one partner is threatening or violent, it greatly increases the odds that the other partner will respond with violence. Sometimes it can be hard to figure out where things started and who started them. But if you can be clear for yourself about what your own role was in the violence, then you will be empowered to make your life safe. This is what we call taking responsibility."

Before each woman shares her story, it is important to explain important guidelines:

- Each woman is to use the victim's first name. This acknowledges him as a human being with a real identity and real feelings—as opposed to an object. When, in our minds, we stop seeing a person as a human being, we are steps closer to making excuses to ourselves for our violence: "If he is a worthless piece of garbage ... then he has no feelings, no value ... and it doesn't matter that I kick or stab him."

- Taking responsibility for one's behavior means not *minimizing*. Examples of minimizing are: "I only pushed him. He exaggerates; it wasn't that bad." What can be especially confusing for a woman is when her male partner minimizes the woman's violence by laughing or taunting. In retelling her story to group, she may also laugh and feel justified in doing so. This warrants a serious response from the therapist and clarification that even if a man laughs or taunts, violence is still violence. Sometimes, however, a woman may laugh because she feels nervous and ashamed to be admitting aloud her bad behavior. The therapist may note that the laughter is confusing because her story sounds very upsetting or alarming, then ask if she means to convey that she thinks the violence was funny. This can be an opportunity to point out that sometimes when our inside emotions are uncomfortable, we try to hide from them with our laughter, but this is dishonest and invalidating of ourselves.

- Taking responsibility means not *blaming*. If a woman frames her violence as justified because someone else or circumstances made her do it, it is helpful to point out: "No one *makes* you kick, or stab, or push. It is a personal choice." We often refer to a sign in the group room that states; "Acknowledge feelings, choose behavior." This can also be an opportunity to ask the women why they think people often blame others for their own behavior (to avoid punishment, to retaliate, to avoid acknowledging one's flaws, to avoid having to take action or change, etc.) and how this ends up working out (feel guilty, blocks closeness and can harm or end relationships, gives power to the other person, can aggravate violence in the relationship).

- Taking responsibility is the opposite of *denial*. Sometimes when a woman starts group, she will acknowledge only a part of her violent behavior, while the police report or report from probation clearly describes many more acts of violence. The therapist may note the discrepancy and ask her about it. If the woman is intractable, this may not be worth arguing about as long as she does take responsibility for something she did do and shows that she wants to learn to behave differently. As women have been in the group longer, they commonly will share that they did more in the original incident than they had first reported, or that while they were arrested for this one incident, they have been even more violent other times and were not arrested for those.

After each woman has shared the story of her violence that led her to this program, she is asked to share with the group some information from her initial homework: her personal goals for this next year, her goals related to the program, her physical cues that tell her she's beginning to get angry, and examples of triggers for this anger. Other group members are asked if they would like to ask her additional questions. They may ask about the domestic violence (Were drugs or alcohol involved? Was she also injured? What is the status of relationship now?) or other topics (Does she have children? What are their ages? Does she have custody or visitation? Does she have a job outside the home or go to school?). Often they will comment on how they identify with what she has experienced or done and commend her for her honesty and forthrightness.

This exercise of sharing helps the women to begin to see that they are part of a community and not alone, that although they have made mistakes, there is hope and they can change.

Women often form positive, meaningful attachments with other group members and want to be able to reach out to each other between group meetings. This can be very constructive and helpful, so the therapist may periodically offer to make a phone list for the group. She passes around a paper with her own name and phone number already written and notes that participation is completely voluntary. "If you write your first name and phone number on this, you are giving me permission to copy it and distribute it to other group members. People may have lots of good reasons to not participate, and no one has to explain what those are. If you do not put your name on the list, I will not give your phone number to anyone else in the group."

When a New Member Joins an Established Group

While some women prefer the intimacy of the smaller initial group and object to the addition of new members, others may feel self-conscious and welcome a larger group where they are less in the spotlight. In any case, adding new members may pose somewhat of a disruption to the dynamics of the group. The most helpful way to ease this transition is to, as much as possible, give notice to the group a week before a new member will be joining. Have current members recall what it was like to attend for the first time and think about what would have made it easier for them. This is now an opportunity for them to reach out to another woman and help her feel accepted and comfortable. Once this informal welcoming happens, it is easier for group members to spontaneously continue on their own as new members join.

When a woman enters an established group, she typically feels anxiety, fear, and shame. (Are the other women going to like me? Will they think I'm a horrible criminal? Will they be scary and tough? Are they going to be cliquish? Will I fit in? Will they be kind and understanding or critical and mean? Is the therapist going to put me on the spot, embarrass me, or tell me how bad I am? Will I be safe here?)

To alleviate this anxiety and integrate the new woman into the group, it is helpful to first have the existing group members introduce themselves to the new member. This exercise is called the newcomer's introduction. Besides easing the new member's anxiety, it also serves as an opportunity for each member to take responsibility for her own behavior without minimizing, denying, or blaming. Going around the circle, each woman introduces herself to the new member by stating her own first name and a one- or two-sentence statement about what she did that landed her in this program. For example: "Hi, Mary. My name is Sam and I'm here because I stabbed my boyfriend, Justin, in the leg with a pen." The statement is simple, clear, and nonshaming, without editorializing. The purpose is taking responsibility.

If a woman does not use her partner's name, this is an opportunity to not only ask her for his name, but also tell the newcomer why this is significant to do. Women, especially early in the program, may frame their statements to defend their violence. The therapist might ask the rest of the group: Is the statement really an example of responsibility? Why not? Did it include minimization, denial, or blame? How could they help her say it more clearly.

The newcomer is then asked to share her story—the whole nine yards, including context and history. When the next newcomer joins, she will be expected to introduce herself as the existing group members have done. She is also asked to share information from her initial homework.

Existing group members are asked if they have questions or comments, and often tell a new woman: "Welcome, that's how I felt...," "This is a good place to be ...," "You'll like it more with time ...," "It helps, I like myself more now, I am doing better in life ...," I didn't want to be here at first, but now I look forward to group ...," "This is time for me ...," "I did this, you can too."

When a Member Completes the Program

The clinical decision that a member is ready to exit the program is made by the therapist outside of group time. Before her last group meeting, the exiting woman will already have completed and turned in her final homework.

Readiness to exit the program is more than simply completing 52 weeks of group and basic program requirements. It signifies that the woman has made substantial progress in her quest to be responsible for herself and live without violence. This personal growth is worthy of recognition and can be a powerful reinforcement and learning experience for the whole group.

Group members often feel attached to senior members whom they admire and respect. Saying goodbye provides a valuable forum to honor a woman's hard work and progress, express mixed feelings of sadness and admiration at her leaving, encourage her continued efforts and commitment to nonviolence, and teach new members.

Also, in many women's childhood histories, important people often left without explanation or goodbyes, leaving the women feeling abandoned, confused, hurt, and angry—and with no means to express and process those feelings. This experience in group can provide an example of how goodbyes happen in healthy relationships.

Because the other women started group after she had first told her extended story, the exiting woman is asked to tell the group what happened in the original domestic violence incident. She is then asked to share—given her knowledge and skills now—what she would do differently in the situation if she could go back and change history: What has she learned? How has she changed? What helped her to make these changes? How is her life different now? What is her commitment to continue these changes? What has the experience of being in this group been like for her? What is it like to be saying goodbye? What wisdom does she want to leave with the group?

Each woman around the circle is then asked to respond individually to the exiting woman. Longer-time group members model for newer members. They may recall a time they laughed together; marvel at how they used to think; thank the woman for her friendship, something specific she taught them, or the example or inspiration she has been. They often share tearfully that knowing this woman has motivated them to do better in life, and that they will miss her in group, even if they intend to continue the friendship outside. They wish her well as she continues her path of nonviolence. Newest members may say that while they do not know her very well, they are encouraged by her example, to know that things can get better, that there is hope.

The Work of the Therapist: Therapist as Teacher

In many ways, the therapist is the consummate teacher. She overtly presents didactic information and teaches specific concepts and skills, and yet, the most powerful and effective learning happens experientially through *how* she teaches.

We want clients to learn the tools of specific skills, but even more so, we want them to *experience* those skills so they can translate and apply them in all of their relationships. We want them to experience a shift in personality, in how they see themselves and others. If a woman changes only superficially (e.g., can use tools but does not change how she sees herself and others), she is at greater risk of being violent again. Permanent change requires deeper healing and does not happen quickly or easily.

External Regulator

The therapist provides external structure so that group members can develop internal structure. She sets the tone for the group experience, establishing safety, trust, and community. She provides safe "holding" of clients' overwhelming emotions and teaches them to manage and regulate them. She shows emotional literacy, self-awareness, and self-responsibility, and helps women define new narratives for how they view themselves and others.

She is a role model. She not only tells them the components of emotional regulation and healthy relationships, but also demonstrates these qualities by her own example.

By providing reparative experiences in group, she helps clients learn empathy for themselves and others. She helps them to recognize the cycle of attachment, attunement, misattunement, and repair as a process they can understand and master. She instills hope that they can have happy satisfying relationships. She is a "good momma."

First: Create a Safe Place

When forming a new group or when a new member joins, women are going to be more reticent about self-disclosing beyond the minimum asked.

The therapist's overriding goal, then, is to create a safe place (safe harbor and secure base) for group members to open up and begin thoughtfully considering the choices they have made in behavior and in life. When a woman says something obviously outrageous, the other group members may snicker, gasp, or freeze. But most of all, they will study the therapist to see how she responds. From her response, they will decide if they are safe in the group.

While it is essential to hold women accountable for their behavior, it is also essential for them to feel understood and supported. This can be an opportunity to introduce the concept of what happens in a healthy family. The therapist may say:

> As we all get to know each other and get closer, we are going to be something like a family. So I want to talk to you about what happens in a healthy family. In a healthy family, each family member *matters*. Each family member is important and worthy of being treating with respect. We are on the same side, we are in this together. No one gets laughed at or belittled. No one is excluded or ignored. Each family member has a right to be heard and listened to. We are here to support and care for each other, and teach each other how to do better in life. So … what this means is that here, in group, every question is worthwhile. This is how everyone learns.

Fostering Community by Building Motivation

It is important to remember that lack of empathy is what sustains the anger response.

Rather than aggressively confronting new members, it is more effective to gently challenge. The therapist may ask a woman to tell more about a situation she is describing and ask the group what questions come to mind that they would like to ask so they can better understand her and her situation. Open-ended questions, reflective listening, and summarizing are all ways of conveying empathy. Asking for more information can also be a useful strategy in de-escalating tension and encouraging self-reflection.

If the woman relaxes and appears willing to further examine her thoughts and feelings, it can be helpful to begin developing the *discrepancy* between what her behaviors have been and what her goals are. Often when women are violent toward a partner, they have not actually considered their immediate goals or their broader, long-term goals. It can be helpful to simply ask the woman what she was hoping she would get by throwing the plate, stabbing her boyfriend, or pushing him down the stairs. Did it get her what she wanted? In the short term? In the long run? In other words, did it work? Even if the woman maintains it got her what she wanted in the short term, she usually can recognize that it was hurtful to someone she cared about and has damaged their relationship. This can then help motivate her to change.

What if, instead, she remains agitated, unwilling to consider her behavior and its consequences? In that case, a good principle to remember is, Roll with resistance and avoid arguments.

If a woman is agitated and defensive, no challenge will effectively change how she is seeing things at that moment. A therapist might simply acknowledge her disagreement, perception, or feeling; thank her for sharing; and then move on. This can demonstrate to group members a helpful strategy for dealing with conflict. Often, women who have been violent have believed that they *must* keep fighting until one side concedes, no matter the damage. This shows them a workable alternative.

If the woman is more directly hostile and challenging toward the therapist, a few different options are worth considering. To "Who are you to tell me what to do? What makes you such an expert?" the therapist might respond: "Well, even though I sometimes like to think I know *something*, I certainly don't know *everything*, and there's probably a lot that I don't know about you and your life. It's probably hard to imagine how I could possibly understand you and what you've been through. Is that right?" To "I can't believe I have to pay for this! The court is just bleeding me dry with all of these fines!" the therapist might respond: "It's hard to have to work hard and pay for this when you don't think you're going to get anything out of it. Is that right?"

Sometimes, this "joining in" is enough to disarm the fight and invite the client to share more about herself. If not, at the very least the group members have the opportunity to observe the therapist staying calm and maintaining a clear sense of herself while being challenged. If she is going to be effective in teaching women these skills, she must have them mastered in her own life.

Beyond Resistance: Early in Group

As it is common at first for women to be reluctant to disclose very personal information or ask for advice, this is a good time to focus group attention on learning specific skills and principles for nonviolence: self awareness, self-responsibility, self-soothing when anxious or distressed, communication, assertiveness, sharing power and control, and so forth.

In the process of discussing these principles, women commonly will start bringing up situations that have stymied them and ask for advice. Always, using their own examples (over the program examples) will be more effective. The more that women bring their own situations to group for discussion, the more they will begin to see the range of alternative approaches for dealing with problems, feel empowered to try them, and believe that change is possible. When this happens, they typically become more motivated to participate in group and to learn.

As Group Coalesces: Weaving Program Concepts

As group members feel more comfortable with the therapist and with each other, they will show more initiative in bringing problems and topics to group because they want help. Beyond concrete problem solving, this often provides many opportunities to explore deeper issues of how women see themselves—in their families, the community, and the culture—and how they became who they are, what faulty beliefs they have carried from childhood about themselves and relationships.

At this point, the therapist has moved from the role of didactic teacher to that of discussion facilitator—speaking less as group members speak more. She must think on her feet, attending to the woman who is speaking as well as the rest of the group as she asks herself:

- What is going on right now individually with this woman?
- What is going on with each other woman and the group as a whole?
- Who is engaged? Who is somewhere else?
- How am I feeling? What is my internal response to what is being shared?
- How can I help the group come together to help the woman who is distressed?
- What do I want to accomplish here? Is the woman headed in the right direction or does a warning alarm need to be sounded for her?

- Which intervention would be most effective? Responding directly with my advice? Asking group members for suggestions based on their experiences or what they have learned? Referring to core principles of the program or a binder handout? Role-playing? Having the group brainstorm problem-solving options? Facilitating a discussion about the underlying issues in the presenting problem?
- Will this choice achieve my expected outcome?

Empowering Without Shaming

The most lasting and valuable knowledge that a woman learns comes from herself, not from the therapist. Women are empowered when they experience that they can make their own choices and decisions for dealing with their lives. The therapist is available for advice but does not give it if the woman does not want it. Timing is critical. Unwanted advice will only fall on deaf ears.

When the woman indicates she does not want any input, the therapist might ask if it is all right to only ask questions to better understand her situation more clearly, yet still respect her request to not be told what to do. Either choice must be respected.

It is important to make it safe for a woman to refuse unwanted feedback, especially when coming from other group members who can be impassioned and overwhelming to a hesitant woman. The opportunity to simply hear one's thoughts aloud without interference can, in and of itself, be a therapeutic process. Asking if a woman wants feedback or would rather just be heard can encourage her to consider what she wants from the group and practice stating it more clearly. The therapist may respond simply with "Thank you for sharing" and move on.

If the woman rebuffs feedback but is clearly in trouble, the therapist may say: "I am really worried for you. I think you are treading in dangerous territory and I don't want to see you get hurt again. When you are ready for advice or input, just give me the sign, let me know. Collectively, when we put the creativity and resources together of all the women in this room, there is impressive wisdom here. We are here for you when you are ready." Then it is time to move on in group.

Allowing a woman to refuse unwanted feedback can be a valuable experience for helping her to feel safe, develop interpersonal boundaries, and recognize that she has a right to say no and is capable of taking care of herself.

When a Woman Does Want Advice

Usually, women who are struggling with difficult situations will want advice, especially if they are comfortable with the therapist and see the group as a helpful resource. Based on her knowledge of the woman, the woman's history, and the time constraints of a group meeting (e.g., number of women who have asked for group time), the therapist may consider different options:

- Respond directly, make specific recommendations and explain the rationale. If the issue has been addressed before in group for this woman or for others, or if time is limited, this might be the most expedient option. For example: "Your ex-husband has a no-contact restraining order against you, not the other way around, right? Even though it's not appropriate for him to be text-messaging and calling you, you miss him and wish you could be together. But you need to think about your own safety and welfare. If you text him back or call him, you are the one who could be in trouble, not him. Do you want to risk that?"
- Ask the group if anyone would like to respond. Women will often place greater value on advice from others who have been in their circumstances than on what the therapist may recommend. Women might remind each other of things they have tried in the past and the results. "Remember how my boyfriend kept calling me and leaving me those threatening messages? The one time I picked up the phone and yelled back at him, he said I was abusing him and that he was going to call my P.O. It was a big mess. I thought if I talked to him and explained things, he'd understand. But it didn't work. I got really mad at him and blew up. I still have feelings for him and I think he does for me. But I can't risk getting in trouble and I'd also hate to see you get in trouble. If your boyfriend really cares about you, he will be respectful toward you. He can follow the restraining order he got, or he can get it modified so you are safe to talk to him. In the meantime, I wish you'd screen all your calls and tell your P.O. what's going on. Your safety is most important. You could also think about getting a restraining order so he can't do that to you."
- Ask the group what questions they have. If not enough questions are asked when a problem is presented, advice may be premature or flawed. Finding out more information slows down the process, de-escalates anxiety, and facilitates women being more thoughtful and less volatile. They might ask, "What is he saying in his messages? Why does he want to talk to you? Does he sound like he's drunk or high? When you get a message from him, how do you feel? Annoyed, nervous, scared, hopeful?

Why are you listening to his messages? Does it make you feel close to him? Is this good for you in the long run or does it hurt you?"

- Ask the woman what she would like the eventual outcome to be after this immediate situation. "Do you think this is possible or likely, given the facts you are sharing with us right now? What would have to change to accomplish your goal? In what ways would he have to change? How would you have to do things differently? What do you have control over? What are you powerless over? If he does not change, what will that mean for you? Is there anything you'd like to make a commitment to doing differently, given all of this?"

When a Woman Discloses Her Aggressive Behavior

An essential part of the therapeutic experience is for women to feel safe in disclosing their ongoing experiences and failures so they can ultimately better understand themselves and learn from mistakes. The newer they are to group, the more anxious and vulnerable they are likely to feel when telling the group about times they have fallen short.

Rarely do women behave badly on purpose. Typically, they start out with good intentions and in spite of themselves, get derailed along the way. When a woman is able to tell the group her regrets about her behavior, she is likely to feel anxious and may appear either defensive, hostile, or tearful. This is an opportunity to appeal to the best in her and acknowledge the part of her that wants to change.

The therapist might say: "That really takes a lot of courage to open up to the group like you just have. Thank you. I'm wondering if it would be all right for us to talk with you more so we can sort out what happened and where you think you got yourself off track. That way, we can help you and everyone else can learn from your experience and your courage in speaking up. Would that be OK?"

If a woman says no, then that must be respected. She may need to calm down before she will be able to thoughtfully discuss what happened. The therapist can reassure her that if she changes her mind, the group still wants to be helpful to her.

When she says yes, the therapist can ask her to slow down the story, start from the beginning and tell what she was thinking, feeling, and doing at each step. For example:

Client 1: I was really excited because my husband had said he was coming home early from work and we could spend the evening together. I cooked all afternoon and made his favorite dinner—pot roast and twice-baked potatoes. I thought about how much I love him and how nice this was going to be for us. Money is so tight, we hardly ever get to go out ... so this was going to be a treat. I even arranged for the kids to go to a friend's so we could be alone.

Therapist: You were looking forward to a special evening alone with him?

Client 1: Yes. I told myself this will bring us closer to each other and repair some of the damage we've been through.

Therapist: Then what happened?

Client 1: I cleaned up, changed into his favorite dress, and lit candles around the house. I had soft music playing in the background. I thought: This is really going to be nice!

Therapist: You put a lot of effort into setting the stage for a nice evening. You sound like you were proud of yourself.

Client 1: Yes, I was! I felt like I was really trying hard. Things have been so bad between us since my arrest that I wanted to show him that it could be like the old days when we first fell in love.

Therapist: You had noble intentions.

Client 1: I did!

Therapist: What happened next?

Client 1: I waited and waited for him to come home, but he didn't show up. I tried to distract myself with TV or a magazine, but it didn't work. After a half hour, I called his cell phone but he didn't pick up. So, I left a message asking him to call me.

Therapist: What were your thoughts then? What were you telling yourself?

Client 1: Well ... as more minutes ticked by, my mind started racing faster and faster. At first I told myself he probably got stuck in traffic and was just running late. Or maybe he forgot to turn on his cell phone—he can be so absent-minded. I wondered if he was OK. I turned on the radio to see if there was an accident ... maybe he was hurt ... or even in the ditch ... or dead! I wondered: Will the police call me or come out to the house? What would I do? How would I support myself and the kids on what I make? Before you know it, I had his funeral planned plus the whole rest of my life without him. Then I started remembering that woman he works with who had flirted with him at his Christmas Party. Maybe they went out for drinks after work! The cheat! How could he do this to me!

Therapist: This is beginning to sound like you were making a motion picture in your head.

Client 1: I totally was! I was creating a whole story line to explain to myself why he wasn't home yet.

Therapist: What were you doing when you were creating the story? How you were feeling—physically and emotionally?

Client 1: Well … I kept pacing back and forth in our house. The more I tried to figure things out, the worse I felt. My stomach was in knots and my head was starting to pound. I went outside and sat on the swing, trying to regroup.

Therapist: You were trying to take care of yourself and calm down?

Client 1: Yes, but it wasn't working. I couldn't figure out if I was more *worried* or more *angry* with him.

Therapist: You sound like you might have been scared.

Client 1: Hmm … well, yes … now that I think about it, fear *was* the biggest feeling I had underneath it all. I was terrified I was losing him. But it was too scary to admit it to myself … it was easier to be angry.

Therapist: That can be a pretty overwhelming feeling to have, that kind of terror, fear.

Client 1: [*Thoughtful*] In retrospect, I think it was so awful an emotion that I ended up doing that thing you call "a blanket of anger to cover the pain."

Therapist: Instead of acknowledging your real feelings, you hid them under the anger?

Client 1: Yes. The more I called his cell phone and he didn't answer, the angrier I got. I was telling myself: Here we go again. I'm trying hard to make things nice and he doesn't even bother to show up! How could he do this to me? I have never cheated on him, so how dare he cheat on me?

Therapist: You had quite a tailspin going. So, how did the motion picture work out?

Client 1: I was a wreck! I started opening up all the kitchen cupboards to see if there was any wine that we'd missed when we threw it all out. I just wanted to calm my nerves. I was pulling out cans and bottles of everything and throwing them on the floor.

Therapist: You were feeling pretty desperate by then?

Client 1: I was totally undone. My hair was a mess and my dress was torn. I was standing on the counter with my head in the back of the cupboard when he finally came home.

Therapist: Wow! What happened then?

Client 1: Well … deep down inside I was relieved to see him and know that he was OK. But I was also *livid* that he was alive and hadn't even called me! I didn't even give him a chance to talk. I had a bottle of horseradish in my hand, so I threw it at him and screamed, "F— you!" Fortunately, he ducked, so it missed him. I was sobbing and ran into the back bedroom. When I first started this program, we made an agreement about how we're going to handle bad times and that when I need to take a time-out, he needs to leave me alone. So, that's what we did.

Therapist: How are things now?

Client 1: Well … I've calmed down some and I told him I'm really, really, really sorry. He's acting pretty standoffish with me. I think he thinks I'm crazy. Plus he knew I was looking for alcohol.

Therapist: Did you find any?

Client 1: No. And I'm glad I didn't. That really would have made things worse.

Therapist: So you've been able to talk with each other?

Client 1: Yes … I found out that he was late because his boss told him to finish up a big project that he wasn't planning on. He thought he'd just be a little late getting home, so he didn't call when he left work, but then he got stuck in traffic. He didn't answer his cell phone because the battery was dead. He hadn't been with the woman from work at all.

Therapist: Hmm … Your motion picture turned out to not be true at all.

Client 1: No. All it did was make me feel more helpless and more afraid.

Therapist: And you had such good intentions. You really wanted to make this a wonderful evening for the two of you.

Client 1: I did, but now I think they're worse than ever.

Therapist: Well, the interesting thing about situations like this is how quickly they can unravel before our very eyes. First off, I really want to give you a lot of credit for coming clean with the group about what you did. That shows a lot of courage and, actually, even integrity. Taking responsibility for your own behavior is the first step in getting better. You can't change what has already happened, but maybe we can take a look at this and learn something helpful. OK?

Client 1: OK … I want to hear what everybody has to say.

[Several group members raise hands to speak. The therapist calls on each individually.]

Client 2: Well, I just want to say: Next time, call me! I love pot roast and twice-baked potatoes, and I'll be over in a flash! [*The group's laughter eases the tension.*]

Client 3: I totally know what you felt like when he wasn't home on time. My boyfriend is always late, and it's hard to handle when you are trying so hard on your part. We all know you love him and that had to be such a letdown for you to have worked so hard to make this a special event.

Client 1: It ended up being "special," but not in the way I wanted it to.

Client 4: I think you need to give yourself some credit here. You did make some mistakes, but you also did some things right.

Therapist *(to client 1):* Can you see what things you did that were right?

Client 1: Well ... I started out with good intentions. I had a worthy goal— to create a nice evening together. I didn't *want* to hurt him.

Client 5: I think you did some other right things. It sounds like you could tell that you were getting upset, so you went outside to the swing, to try to calm down.

Client 6: Plus, even though you threw the horseradish, you realized that wasn't OK and you didn't keep making things worse. That was good that you and your husband had the time-out agreement and that you followed it.

Client 1: I guess I just wish I could go back and undo things.

Therapist: Well, let's take a look at that—the first step that you wish you hadn't taken. Where do you think that was?

Client 1: I think it was when I started making the motion picture. I was trying to figure out what had happened, but all the things I told myself made me feel worse and worse.

Therapist: What do you wish you hadn't done?

Client 1: I think I wish I had not made such a mess by throwing everything out of the cupboards. I just had to clean it up the next day. But even more, I wish I hadn't thrown the horseradish ... I could have really hurt my husband and I don't want to do that. I wish I hadn't used profanity. Freaking out isn't going to change whatever the reality is. I love him, but I didn't treat him in a loving way. The idea of losing him is so terrifying that sometimes it's hard to imagine that I'd even be able to breathe. I think he feels like he walks on eggshells around me, and I don't want him to feel like that.

Therapist: Those are hard things to admit to, but it is impressive that you have such a clear vision of what you wish you had *not* done. Can you think of what you wish you *had* done instead?

Client 1: Well, I hope there never is a next time, but I'd like to be able to stay calm when I don't know where he is. It would have been so cool if he could have walked in to me relaxing on the sofa ... we could have gone ahead and had a wonderful evening together.

Therapist: What are some things you could do to be able to stay calm and relax on the sofa?

Client 1: Well, I *was* kind of tired out from getting ready. It would have been hard, but I could have lain down on the sofa and listened to the music I was playing. If that didn't work, I could have called up someone else from group for some support and reassurance, so I wouldn't feel so alone. I could remind myself that my husband and I been through a lot and we're still together. Whatever might be going on, *I* can survive and *we* can survive.

Therapist: That sounds like a good plan. How are you feeling inside right now?

Client 1: [*Pausing*] A lot calmer, quieter, more at peace. It really helped to be able to talk about it. Thank you all for listening and being here for me.

Because we are most receptive to difficult answers when we come upon them ourselves, a woman's own understanding and solutions will always be her most effective instruction. The therapist, then, takes a supportive role, guiding her to their discovery.

Therapist Self-Disclosure and Use of Self

An interesting aspect of this work is how it forces us as therapists to take stock of ourselves and how we manage our own personal lives. As we listen to women's stories in group, we cannot help but hear an inner dialog that asks what we would do in the same circumstances. Through our everyday life experiences and our closest relationships, we will be confronted with our insecurities, challenges, and failures. To be truly effective in helping women with their violence, we must have the courage to confront our own.

While some women will idealize the therapist and revere whatever she says, others will search for her Achilles' heel and work to expose her every weakness. She must strike a delicate balance between her expertise and competence, and her awareness of her vulnerability. She must be clearly in charge and responsible for the integrity of the therapeutic experience of the group and program, and yet still be human.

Authenticity

The strongest therapeutic relationship is possible when the therapist is consciously aware of her own internal thoughts and feelings and uses this as helpful additional information to better understand clients—individually and as part of the group process. Women referred to this type of group often are hypervigilant to any indication that the therapist is frustrated, angry, bored, anxious, tense, and so forth. Just because they sense this does not mean they will ask about it, however.

I have found it helpful when I sense tension in the group to say so, and ask if anyone else is sensing it. Sometimes the tension will have to do with drama between group members, sometimes with individual member's crisis, and sometimes with group members' perceptions of the therapist. In any case, it is important to make the unspoken, spoken—to put the issue on the table so it can be addressed and, if necessary, resolved. All of this is useful "grist for the mill."

Because so many women grew up in families where adults never explained their own behavior or what was happening in the family, this can be an opportunity for the therapist to model authenticity and humility. If the tension is about her, this can be a valuable opportunity for the therapist to invite and listen to group members' perceptions of her. It does not mean that she will always fully answer every question, but it can help her understand how the women see her.

Humility

It is appropriate and instructive for the therapist to acknowledge that she does not know everything. In fact, some things she will never know as well as the clients will know. For instance, she will never know their own internal experiences, thoughts, and feelings as well as they do. When she makes a mistake, her willingness to acknowledge this, apologize, and work toward repair will provide a powerful example of what we want clients to learn. This can be a good time to remind herself to view a client's criticism as constructive feedback that will help her do even better—rather than taking it personally.

Monitoring Countertransference

Sometimes, interactions with clients may arouse within the therapist primitive feelings of rage, terror, helplessness, or other equally distressing emotions. Especially with women with borderline personality disorder, the therapist may find herself doubting her clinical skills and questioning whether she can ever do anything right. Unexamined, the therapist's countertransference can interfere with treatment and, at its worst, harm the client.

It is absolutely essential that the therapist have access to regular consultation with colleagues to debrief and sort out which issues are her client's and which are her own. If she has unresolved issues in her history or current life, it is imperative that she seek her own psychotherapy to address these so that they do not unwittingly affect her work with the group.

Self-Disclosure

As women are in group longer and feel more comfortable with the therapist, they may ask her personal questions. Even if women have not verbalized the questions, I believe that they have them inside, and that it is better to hear them and be able to discuss them, than to flatly refuse them.

Before answering any question, though, it is important to understand the motivations behind them. Some questions come from simple curiosity and wanting to know the therapist better as a person. Other times, the questions are really asking: Do you know what you are talking about? Do you have anything of value to teach me? Have you ever struggled and survived? How did you do it? Can I trust you or will you betray me? Do you care about me? Can you understand me?

When done thoughtfully and carefully, I believe that self-disclosure can be helpful in deepening the therapeutic alliance. Always, the therapist must be certain that whatever she is disclosing is to benefit the client.

When clients have asked about my personal life, I have told them that I am married and have two children who are now grown. Sometimes, when wanting to illustrate a particular concept or skill, I will use an example from my own life.

For instance, one week when I wanted to explain how to do the ongoing journal homework, I started group by telling the women that I had just learned something important about myself and would like to share it with them. I told them that at first it was hard to admit it to myself and that I felt kind of embarrassed. The room became very quiet, and this is what I told them:

> After a rocky adolescence when my daughter and I seemed to be butting heads on every front, she and I have finally worked things out and are very close. We talk lots, we laugh, she tells me all about her life and even asks me for advice! (You can imagine what a thrill that is for me!)
>
> Well, she's 24 and has recently fallen in love with a wonderful man and they plan to marry. This last weekend, she met his parents for the first time. She told me how they really hit it off. Like me, her future mother-in-law is also a clinical social worker. They stayed up late at night and talked all weekend about families, relationships, and intimate secrets—*the very things I talk with my daughter about.*
>
> So, as she was telling me this, I was getting a knot in my stomach and starting to choke up. I said the right things, but when I hung up the phone I was feeling kind of sick. I was thinking: *What if Meredith likes her better than me?* I felt displaced, excluded, and jealous ... hard things to have to admit.

The group responded sympathetically and told me how awful this was. One suggested I set the record straight with my daughter, and another said I'd better tell her not to call her in-laws mom and dad. I said:

> This was hard, but as I sat with myself and thought about it, I realized that what was going on inside of me was about me, not my daughter. I was feeling tied up because of how I was *choosing* to look at the situation. The more I thought about it, I could see that I *want* my daughter to have a good relationship with her mother-in-law. That can make her life a lot easier and be better for her marriage. I know my daughter loves me and I love her. I will always be her mom and she will always be my daughter. I have enough love for more than one child, so I'm sure she can have enough love for more than one mother.

My willingness to self-disclose and be vulnerable prompted other group members to share about their own family experiences and times they had felt jealous and left out. Some spoke up more personally and passionately than they had ever done before in group. We talked about how perception can create feelings of jealousy, how to cope with hurt feelings, and the value of finding compassion for ourselves and others.

I believe our discussion was far more meaningful and memorable for the group members than if I had only asked them to open their binders to the homework page and read through each step of doing a journal entry. In this discussion, they were able to connect personally and emotionally to the material, and thereby learn more from the experience.

10

Using Binder Handouts to Facilitate Growth and Change

When a treatment program is designed and certified to accept court-ordered domestic violence offenders, the state will determine the length of the program. This varies from state to state. The program described in this book is designed to comply with California state law, which mandates 52 weeks of treatment.

Although some states allow a shorter term of treatment, my personal opinion is the longer, the better. Shorter programs can teach specific skills but do not have the necessary time to address the deeper wounds of childhood abuse and trauma that so many of these women carry with them—and that have set the stage for their adult relationship violence. Many have little self-awareness or sense of self and often have poor boundaries. These are all issues for which there is no authentic quick fix.

When a program must be shorter (e.g., 12 to 16 weeks), the priority is to cover the information in Sections 2 and 3 of the binder. When a program is somewhat longer (e.g., 16 to 26 weeks), Section 4 can be covered. Section 5 (family of origin) is for the longest programs.

Because group enrollment is open-ended, women will be discussing issues at different stages of their participation in the program. It is up to the therapist to use her judgment in deciding the focus of each group meeting. Where one group meeting ends will invariably suggest where the next should start.

This chapter will provide recommendations for facilitating groups, and then suggestions for introducing and discussing specific topics (corresponding to specific binder handouts). Not all binder handouts are discussed below because simply reading them with the group will generate enough discussion and reflection.

General Recommendations

We all learn best when we are able to relate content to our own life experiences. When women are newer to group, they may be more reticent to self-disclose. For those times, it can be helpful to use the hypothetical examples provided as a springboard for discussion. Ideally, however, discussions will draw out the women's personal stories, which can then be explored. Always, priority is given to group member's stories and experiences. Content and principles can then be woven through discussion of these.

We also learn best from repetition. When introducing a topic, it is valuable to state the objectives clearly and explicitly: "This is what we are going to be talking about, and this is why I think it's important for you to get it." When addressing a topic that has been discussed previously, start with a review: "What do you remember about ...? Why is this important?"

A fundamental recurring theme is the concept of a healthy family. One of the therapist's tasks is to create a group experience that models a healthy family. This can be stated explicitly and implicitly throughout the course of the program. The therapist can tell the group that this is her goal—for each woman to experience what happens in a healthy family—and then ask: "What happens in a healthy family?"

The answer is:

- Everyone feels safe and is safe.
- Each person is valued as important and essential to the family.
- Each person feels connected to the family—a sense of belonging.
- Each person has a voice, is listened to, and is treated with respect.
- Each person's thoughts, feelings, and opinions matter.
- The family works together to help and support each member—even when issues are not resolvable.
- Boundaries are respected.
- The family members do not keep secrets about trauma that family members have experienced. The family talks about what has happened and changes to safeguard the safety of the members.

Section 1 Binder Contents: Policies and Rules

Suggestions to Therapist: Group Rules

This handout addresses essential boundaries for the group. It is worth reviewing in group every so often as a reminder. After each rule is read, the therapist may ask: "Why do you think this is an important rule to have here?"

Handout: Group Rules

1. Safety for *all* is the priority.
2. Be on time to group and prepared to participate and learn.
3. Turn off cell phones.
4. Respect confidentiality. If you share information outside of group, focus on topics discussed and your own experiences. *Do not* disclose any group members' names or identifying information.
5. Give the speaker your full attention. If you want to ask a question or speak, raise your hand and wait to be called on.
6. Speak respectfully. No swearing or cursing. Racist, sexist, and homophobic remarks are inappropriate and will not be tolerated.
7. If you find yourself feeling upset when someone else in group is sharing, ask yourself: What does this trigger inside of me? What are my physical cues right now? My emotions? What is this telling me about myself? What can I learn to help me in my life?

Section 2 Binder Contents: Domestic Violence

Suggestions to Therapist: Ten Truths

This handout can be read at the beginning of the group. The statements summarize key principles of this program. As women have been in the program longer, they may reflect on which statement most speaks to them, which has been most helpful, which they disagreed with, why, and how they think now.

Handout: Ten Truths

1. I am responsible for my own behavior.
2. I am powerless over the thoughts, feelings, and behaviors of others.
3. I am powerless over others, but I am not helpless.
4. I am not to blame if I am hurt, but I *am* responsible to take care of myself and heal my hurt.
5. Anger is a legitimate emotion.
6. I can acknowledge my emotions and choose how I will express them.
7. I can't change my past, but I *can* change my future.
8. Both men and women are worthy of respectful treatment.
9. One act of abuse never justifies another.
10. Violence is *never* an acceptable solution to problems.

Suggestions to Therapist: Domestic Violence:
The Expanded Definition

When asked what they think domestic violence is, most people will answer: "physically hurting someone else." This expanded definition is important because it describes a range of behaviors that are hurtful, intimidating, and abusive and can help women think about how they have treated partners and vice versa. While it may seem obvious, many men and women arrested for domestic violence really do not know the difference between appropriate, acceptable, respectful behavior and inappropriate, hurtful, abusive behavior.

- **Ask:** What do you see on this page that describes how you have been treated? What was the impact on you? What do you see on this page that describes how you have behaved? What do you think has been the impact on your partner? On yourself? Your feelings about yourself?
- It is important for women to have some understanding of *why* they have behaved as they have. Counselor and author Steven Stosny (1995) says that control and abuse in a relationship start with core hurts and a failure of compassion. We hurt people we love when we feel unloveable and because they remind us of the darkest "truths" about ourselves. We mislead ourselves into thinking we can relieve our pain by manipulating our attachment figures. In the history of human kind, has anyone ever felt more lovable by hurting someone she loves?
- **Ask:** Why do you think women are violent? What do you think motivates women to domestic violence? What do you think of Stosny's explanation? How does this apply to your circumstances, your relationship?

Handout: Domestic Violence: The Expanded Definition

Domestic violence is the use of power to punish, dominate, or control an intimate partner. This can be in the form of physical violence, emotional abuse, sexual abuse, financial abuse, isolation, threats, intimidation, and maltreatment of children.

Physical violence is angry body contact or persistent unwanted body contact that causes direct injury or results in secondary injury; any touch of a person's body with the intent of causing fear. *Examples:* poking, slapping, kicking, hitting, pushing.

Emotional/psychological abuse is non-body contact such as intimidation, threats, gestures, humiliation, name calling, derogatory remarks, or accusations designed to reduce self-esteem. Once physical violence has occurred, emotional abuse has a much more devastating effect, like being held hostage, living in fear. *Examples:* displaying weapons, controlling what a partner does/who he talks to/where he goes, using jealousy to justify actions, threatening to hurt or kill a partner, threatening to leave or commit suicide, using the courts or probation to intimidate or control.

Sexual violence is any sexual act that is forced, coerced, or done under implied threat; continuance of any sex act when consent has been or has become unclear.

Destruction of property is breaking things, throwing things, destroying one's own or another's possessions, assaulting pets. The implication is "you could be next."

Financial abuse is withholding money, secretly taking a partner's money, refusing to buy necessities, secretly spending large sums of money as a means of control, out of anger, or to make a point.

Stalking is following, spying on, threatening, making repeated phone calls, coming to the victim's place of employment, leaving written messages or objects, vandalizing the victim's property. **Cyberstalking** is the use of the Internet and other forms of electronic communications to harass or threaten. *Examples:* harassment in live chat rooms, using the victim's code name or e-mail address after leaving inappropriate messages on message boards or guest books, sending viruses, electronic identity theft.

Racial/ethnic/gender/religious prejudice is bigotry against others because of their race, ethnicity, gender, identity, sexual orientation, or religion. This includes joking and making degrading references to others.

Using female privilege is treating a male partner like a servant, making all the decisions in matters of child care and homemaking, assuming that the man knows nothing, that the woman knows better and should not be questioned.

Using male privilege is treating a female partner like a servant, making all the big decisions, acting like the "master of the castle," being the one to unilaterally determine men's and women's roles.

Suggestions to Therapist: Responsibility and Empowerment

If a woman comes to the program by court order, she has probably heard many times that she must take responsibility for her behavior. Most think they do, but also feel significant shame. "Taking responsibility" is more than the ability to list one's illegal behaviors. Have the group read the handout below.

- **Ask:** Do you agree that responsibility is empowering? Why or why not? Have you ever done something wrong that you didn't get caught for, then owned up to it? How did you take responsibility? What was that like? What happened? Do you regret taking responsibility or are you glad you did? What did you conclude from the experience?
- **Ask:** Was power a factor in the incident that landed you here? How?

Handout: Responsibility and Empowerment

"I am responsible for my own behavior."

What does that mean? It means being really honest with myself, taking time to thoughtfully accept that *I have made choices* for dealing with problems. This is not always an easy thing to do. It takes courage.

Circumstances and relationships can be really complicated. Sometimes, violence is so entrenched in a relationship, that it is nearly impossible to tell where it all started and who was originally responsible. No matter what my partner's behavior has been, I have *chosen* whether I will respond and how I will respond. If my partner is violent, I make a choice to respond with violence or not. No one has made me do anything. I am in charge of myself. I am responsible.

Taking responsibility for my behavior means that I am accountable. I face what I have done without minimizing ("It was only..."), denying ("He may have a black eye, but it's not my fault"), or blaming ("He deserved it ... if he hadn't hurt me, I wouldn't have hurt him"). When I do any of these, I am giving up my power to my partner. I am saying he controls me; I am saying that I am a victim and helpless. There is nothing I can do.

Why is taking responsibility important?

Taking responsibility for my behavior is the first step in my healing. When I take full responsibility for myself and my behavior, *I am empowered* to choose who I am and how I want to live. I am not responsible for my partner's behavior; he chooses that himself. I am only responsible for me.

I recognize what I have control over: myself, my thoughts, feelings, and behavior—and what I have no control over: others and their thoughts, feelings, and behaviors.

The more I take responsibility for myself, the more I have control over my life. I acknowledge myself when I make good choices. I learn from my mistakes. I am kind to myself.

What am I happy with in my life? What would I like to be different? What can I do today?

Suggestions to Therapist: Comparing Relationships:
Equality Versus Power and Control

The handout below can be simply read and discussed in group: To prompt reflection, the therapist may ask the following questions:

- With which parts do you agree and find to be true in your life?
- With which parts do you disagree?
- What parts seem really difficult—or even impossible—to follow? Why?
- If you were able to live according to these principles, how do you think this would affect your life? Your relationship? Your children?

HANDOUT: COMPARING RELATIONSHIPS: EQUALITY VERSUS POWER AND CONTROL

Equality: Power and Control Are Shared	When Power and Control Are Abused
Trust: We are honest and open with each other. We are safe with each other's most vulnerable feelings. We keep each other's confidences.	**Mistrust:** It is not safe for us to be open and honest with each other. If one opens up and is vulnerable, he/she risks being belittled, demeaned, humiliated, or hurt.
Respect: We value each other. We have each other's best interests at heart. We treat each other with care—alone and in front of others.	**Contempt:** We use intimidation, coercion, threats, and manipulation to get what we want from each other. We are quick to criticize and point out flaws.
Responsibility: When either of us makes a mistake, we own up to it. We apologize and reach out to repair the relationship.	**Minimization, denial, and blame:** When one of us hurts the other, we shift responsibility onto the other person. Damage in our relationship is rarely or never repaired.
Decisions are made together: We share power and control. When we make decisions, we have equal voices, equal say in what we decide.	**Decisions are made unilaterally:** Either one partner has all the power and makes all the big decisions, or we fight back and forth in power struggles.
Partnership: We are on the same side. There is a sense of "we-ness." We look for win–win in all situations.	**Adversaries:** There are always two sides with us—one partner wins and one partner loses.
Reliable: We are consistent and predictable with each other. We keep our word. We demonstrate integrity with each other. We can count on each other.	**Unreliable:** If we make promises to each other, sometimes we keep them but often we don't. One or both of us lack integrity. It's better to keep a partner guessing. This feels powerful.
Validation and support: We affirm and celebrate each other's successes. We support each other's strivings to pursue individual interests and hobbies.	**Invalidation:** One partner's competence is seen as a threat to the relationship. The other undermines this success either overtly through words or covertly through body language.
Safety: We value each other's and our safety. Violence in our relationship is untenable.	**Dangerousness:** One of both of us would do whatever it takes to get his/her own way. Violence is seen as a viable option.

Suggestions to Therapist: Am I Safe?

Often, women in group have never considered whether or not their relationships are safe—unless it is in the moments during or after domestic violence.

This handout is designed to help them consider what safety means, how they know they are safe or not, and how they can take responsibility for safety. It also provides useful information that may be referred to as women share dangerous situations in their lives in group.

The therapist may ask: "Has anyone answered these questions for herself? Would you be willing to share with the group?"

Handout: Am I Safe?

Safety is important from two perspectives: my partner's risk and my risk of violence.

- **Is my partner at risk of being violent toward me or my children?**

    The best predictor of future violence is past violence. A person who has an established history of physical, psychological, or sexual violence toward a partner is likely to continue that violence unless there is significant intervention directed at changing the behavior. The greater the following, the greater the risk of harm to victims: history and frequency of violence, severity of injuries, threats to kill, fantasies of homicide or suicide, access to weapons, frequency of drug and/or alcohol use, "ownership" of the partner ("You belong to me forever!"), centrality of the partner (idolizing and depending on partner to organize and sustain the other; if a partner leaves, the other feels justified in retaliating with violence because of the perceived betrayal), disregard or contempt for authority, and recent stressors in life.

    - Is my partner committed to nonviolence in our relationship?
    - Has my partner ever threatened, been violent, or abusive in any way toward me or toward a previous partner? Toward any children?
    - Has my partner ever been arrested or charged with domestic violence? Child abuse?
    - What is my partner's attitude about these charges? Does he take responsibility for his behavior? Did he get help? What is his attitude about getting help? Does he have a support system that helps him stay accountable for his behavior?
    - If I feel threatened, who are the friends, relatives, or agencies I can call in an emergency?
    - If I feel threatened, what safe places can I go to with my children? What is my safety plan? Have I talked about this with my therapist and with the group?

    Note: If you are in an abusive relationship, it is imperative that you take seriously your safety and that of your children's.

- **Am I at risk of being violent to my partner or my children?**
    It is also imperative that you take responsibility for your own behavior. Recognize that no matter how badly your partner may behave, nothing justifies retaliating with violence or abuse. In fact, women who retaliate with violence significantly increase the chances that they will incur worse injuries from their partners.

    - Am I committed to nonviolence in all of my relationships?
    - Do I know my physical cues that tell me I am getting angry or overwhelmed?
    - Do I practice tranquility breathing? Do I take time-outs?
    - Do I call my therapist or other group members when I feel like I'm losing it?
    - Do I ask for help? Do I accept feedback without defensiveness?
    - Do I work on learning from my mistakes?

*Suggestions to Therapist: Physical Cues: The
Brain and the Anger Response*

When we are upset and experiencing our physical cues, our brain has signaled to our entire body the message: "Danger! Alert!" When it is a bona fide emergency, we want to be able to spring into action immediately, without stopping to think. But sometimes our brain is sending out the emergency signals and it is not an imminent life-or-death emergency. With the group, review the binder handout on this topic.

- **Tell the story:** Imagine living in caveman days, tending your children as you cook the family meal over a fire. It's a pleasant, sunny day, the children are happily entertaining themselves, and your husband is off hunting for tomorrow's food.
- Suddenly, a saber-toothed tiger jumps from behind a cluster of bushes and growls at your children, poised to devour any one of them. As the mom, you want to automatically spring into action to save your children and yourself—but this is not the time to think! Thankfully, your amygdala has turned on before you consciously realized you needed it; you have instant, superhuman strength.
- Without thinking, you grab a blazing log from the fire, swing the log in the tiger's face as you match his roars and chase after him—at lightning speed. The tiger, whiskers singed, slinks away to a faraway wilderness. As you return to your children, you realize that your hand has been badly burned by the flaming log.
- Your children hug you, tell you how brave you are, thank you for saving their lives, put grease on your burned hand, and wrap it in leaves. Everything seems to have settled down to a relaxing afternoon when you hear the crackling of leaves near your camp—surge of adrenaline, fight or flight—it is your husband dragging home tomorrow's food.
- **Ask:** How can you tell that your amygdala is activated? What is good about this? What can be problematic about this? Can you think of examples in your life where your amygdala was activated? What happened? How did things work out?
- **Ask:** How long did it take for your prefrontal cortex to kick in? How could you tell? What was it like? What happened?

Handout: Physical Cues: The Brain and the Anger Response

Two parts of the brain are significant to our experience of anger: the amygdala and the prefrontal cortex.

The *amygdala* is a tiny, almond-shaped structure located deep in the middle of the brain. This region of the brain is sometimes referred to as the primitive brain. The amygdala is essential to basic survival and houses our fight-or-flight response. It is either on or off, all or nothing. When activated, it instantly precipitates a cascade of chemicals into the bloodstream (cortisol, epinephrine, and norepinephrine) that increases heart rate, elevates blood pressure, dilates the eyes, stops digestion, tenses muscles, produces a surge of monumental energy, and numbs pain. It focuses the entire body on fighting for survival or running like crazy to escape certain death.

Anger originates in the amygdala and is the only emotion that can activate every muscle group and every organ in the body. While this process is essential for our survival, the amygdala does not distinguish between truly dangerous situations and ones that might be only mildly annoying, or even benign.

That is the job of the *prefrontal cortex.* This structure is located roughly behind the forehead in the region sometimes referred to as the smart brain or thinking brain. The prefrontal cortex operates executive functions: reality testing, judgment, perception, and problem solving. This part of our brain helps us think things through: identify problems, judge the severity of the problems, recognize options, imagine possible corresponding outcomes, and make choices before we act.

Have you ever heard someone described as so angry she couldn't think straight? When the amygdala is activated (on), the prefrontal cortex is out of commission. If the prefrontal cortex is going to work, the amygdala must be off.

How is this relevant to domestic violence? In several ways:

- We experience our *physical cues* that tell us we are angry *before* we have *cognitive recognition* of anger.
- If those physical cues happen during an argument with a partner, we are not going to be able to think clearly until the physical cues subside. We will not be able to listen effectively, negotiate, express ourselves respectfully, or use good judgment. Our perception may be inaccurate, and we may misinterpret our partner's words, behavior, or intentions. We risk making bad choices.
- When we practice self-awareness, we can recognize our physical cues as valuable information. They tell us to take a time-out and calm down until we can think straight.
- When our physical cues have subsided, we can return to the discussion and be more effective in expressing ourselves and getting our needs met.

Suggestions to the Therapist: Time-Outs

Time-out is a foundational skill that each women is expected to have practiced often and mastered before completing the program. With the group, read through the time-outs handout.

- **Ask:** Has anyone here ever taken a time-out? Can you tell us what happened? (Point out the elements of time-outs as described in the handout.)
- **Ask:** What did you do during your time-out? How did you calm yourself? What was the effect of the time-out for you, your partner, and your relationship? Did it help? Why, why not?
- Often, women and men will think that they have taken a time-out anytime they walk away. It is important to underscore that getting in a final jab while storming out the door is *not* a time-out.
- **Ask:** How do you know you need to take a time-out? What kinds of physical cues does everyone here experience? What makes it hard to do time-outs?
- Think of your physical cues as being on a scale of intensity 1–10. If the intensity stays at around a 3–4, you might be able to stay calm enough to still think clearly. But when the intensity gets higher, it is more likely you are losing ability to make rational decisions—time to take a time-out; don't wait until it is too late.
- **Ask:** What kinds of things work for each of you—to help you calm down during a time-out?

Handout: Time-outs

Time-out is an important skill for coping with anger, taking care of yourself emotionally, and helping you avoid behavior that you will later regret. The more you practice time-outs, the better you will get and the more you will feel in charge of yourself, your emotions, and your behavior. The purpose is to de-escalate volatile situations, avoid violence, improve safety, and trust in your relationship.

When done correctly, time-outs demonstrate how much you value your partner and your relationship. It is important to review this page when you are calm and share the information with your partner when you are both calm.

A time-out is *not* a weapon against a partner, a tool for avoiding issues important to your partner, or an excuse to go out and party. A time-out *is* an act of love. It demonstrates the message "I care about you and our relationship so much that I don't want to say or do anything that might push you away."

It is not appropriate to tell your partner when you think he needs to take a time-out; it is his job to decide that for himself. Your job is to decide when *you* need a time-out.

These are the steps for a time-out:

1. Be aware of the physical cues you experience when you are getting angry (e.g., racing heart, tense muscles, hotness, headache, stomach in knots, sweaty palms).
2. When you experience these cues, do not swear, raise your voice, or threaten your partner. Don't comment on your partner's behavior; only speak about yourself.
3. Say: "I'm beginning to get angry and I need to take a time-out."
4. Don't storm out. Tell your partner where you will be (a neutral, safe location) and when you will return (not more than an hour).
    "I'm going for a walk [or bike ride or jog or the gym, or to soak in the bathtub or sit in the backyard]. I'll be back in a half hour."
5. At the safe, neutral place, practice tranquility breathing and calming self-talk. Do not drink, use drugs, or drive. Do not engage in aggressive behaviors (i.e., punching pillows, throwing rocks, etc.), as these are like rehearsing violence.
6. Use this time to calm your physical cues and think more clearly. After you are calm, ask yourself: What is the most important issue in the argument? Is this something resolvable, or something that is OK to disagree about? Does this need to be decided now, or can it be tabled? What is my overall goal?
7. Keep to your agreement: return on time.
8. Decide with your partner if this is a good time for discussion, if later is better, or if this issue does not need to be resolved.

Remember: Safety is the first priority. A time-out does not need a partner's approval. If your partner blocks your path, sit down where you are and practice being quiet. Practice tranquility breathing and, as soon as possible, escape to a safe place and call 911. Remind yourself: Violence never truly solves problems. Safety is most important.

Suggestions to Therapist: Tranquility Breathing

Especially when a woman has experienced trauma in her history, she may feel like she is in a constant state of alert, ever ready for the imminent disaster. It is as if her amygdala is always on. She may not know what it feels like to be in a state of relaxation.

Deep, slow breathing is one of the simplest, most effective ways to calm physical cues so that the prefrontal cortex can engage.

- **Ask:** Did anyone ever go through a childbirth preparation class using Lamaze or Bradley breathing techniques? What was it like? Did you notice a difference in how you felt during labor and delivery?
- Women are often trained and coached to use special breathing techniques that have been shown to decrease the experience of pain during childbirth. Knowing how to breathe can help you feel better physically and emotionally. It takes little time and no special equipment. (Lead the group through the breathing exercise entitled "Tranquility Breathing.")
- **Ask:** How do you feel now? Can you tell a difference? What was the experience like?
- **Ask** everyone to practice this exercise at least once a day and report back at the next group about their experiences.

Handout: Tranquility Breathing

When we are stressed, anxious, or angry, we breathe differently. Consider these differences:

- Anxious breathing is shallow, rapid, through the mouth, in the upper chest.
- Calm breathing is deep, slow, through the nose, in the belly.

Paying attention to and changing how we breathe is one of the fastest and most effective ways to calm down, feel better, and think more clearly.

Try this:

- Think of your lungs as divided into two chambers, one in your upper chest and one in your belly. You will be breathing in and out of the lower chamber.
- Close your eyes, place your hand on your stomach. As you breathe in, your stomach distends, moving your hand out. As you exhale, your stomach flattens and your hand moves in.
- Breathe in slowly through your nose, extending your stomach as your "lower lung" fills with air, counting to 5 (one-one thousand, two-one thousand, etc.).
- Imagine breathing in clean, soothing, refreshing air.
- Hold for two seconds.
- Exhale slowly through your mouth, to the count of 5. Imagine that as you exhale, your breath is grabbing any tension in your body and pushing it out through your mouth.
- Hold two seconds.
- Repeat 10 times. You have just experienced tranquility breathing.

Section 3 Binder Contents: Homework

Suggestions to Therapist: Journal Homework

This ongoing homework assignment will help women learn to be more self-aware and better able to care for themselves emotionally. It is essential to learn to recognize one's emotions and how best to self-soothe in the moment.

- Anger rarely shows up as a single emotion. Invariably, anger is a response to first feeling hurt. But, it is a lot harder to say, "I feel hurt," than to say "I am angry!"
- When the hurt (or other emotion) gets ignored, pushed down, or hidden, we call this "a blanket of anger covering the pain." The apparently angry person has thrown a cover over the pain so no one will know. This can seem powerful and self-protective, but it isn't. It is dishonest and can confuse or push away the very person you want to care about you. It means that you are not talking about your true feelings and can make it a lot harder for the other person to want to understand you or to help you.
- If you deny your own hurt and pain, it is easier to deny or minimize the hurt and pain you cause others.

Review step by step how to do journal homework. Several pages in the binder provide extra help with this: "How to Do Journal Homework," "Emotions Inventory," "Self-Talk: Inflammatory or Calming," and "Examples of Calming Self-Talk."

Each time that a group members turn in journal homework, it is important for the therapist to read the entry, write comments, and return the next week so that the woman will be able to improve. This allows the therapist to gauge how well the woman understands the program concepts and is using new skills. It also can help the therapist know what is going on in her life that she is not sharing in group. The therapist may write on the homework a suggestion that the woman talk about an entry in group or may speak individually to the woman to follow up on a particular situation.

Periodically throughout the program, a group meeting may be devoted to each woman sharing one of her journal homework entries. This facilitates self-disclosure and allows the group members to help each other understand and master the self-awareness that homework is designed to teach.

Additional Important Concepts

- Anger is a normal human emotion, with good and bad aspects to it. The goal of this program is not to eliminate your anger, but to help you *acknowledge feelings and choose appropriate behavior.*
- Reframing is taking a picture and putting it in a different frame, so what you are seeing looks the same but different. **Ask:** When might this be a useful strategy?
- Making motion pictures (see binder handout for description).
- Thoughts, feelings, and behaviors are connected (Figure 10.1). If you want to feel better, change your thoughts and behaviors.
- **Ask:** Which of these do you think you can control? Which can you choose? How? If you want to change your feelings, what can you do? (Use examples of recent situations group members have shared, or ask someone to volunteer an example from her journal homework.)

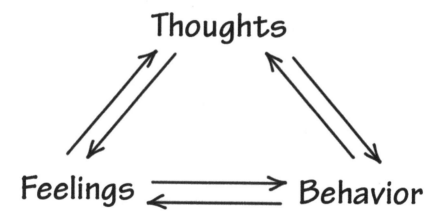

Figure 10.1   Relationship between thoughts, feelings, and behavior.

Handout: How to Do Journal Homework

Journal homework is an important component of this program. Completing homework regularly and thoughtfully will help you to be more self-aware and more empowered to make choices about how you behave. Additional journal homework pages are available at group each week. A minimum of one page (four entries) is due every four weeks.

Practice observing yourself, especially your physical cues that tell you when you are beginning to get upset. Choose one time each week to write about this in your homework. This can be a time you felt angry, or it might be a time you felt any other negative emotion.

1. In the first box, write the date and time of day in which you noticed your physical cues.
2. In the next box, describe the situation. Where were you? What was happening? What were the circumstances? Describe the event behaviorally and use first names of others involved (plus their relationship to you). Do not editorialize—no assuming what someone else's motives are. Simply state others' behavior.
3. Give a number to the intensity of how you were feeling, with 1 as the least intense and 10 as the most intense (i.e., 1 = mild, 10 = explosive).
4. Describe your physical cues (i.e., stomach in knots, ears ringing, muscle tensing, etc.).
5. What emotions—*other than anger*—were you experiencing? (Need help labeling them? Refer to the "Emotions Inventory" page in the binder). Why is this important? This helps you acknowledge the additional and complex emotions that often accompany your anger, or may even be more powerful for you than your anger.
6. Inflammatory self-talk: What did you tell yourself? What were you thinking that would make you feel more angry, heated up, livid?
7. Calming self-talk: What did you tell yourself that helped you to calm down, see the bigger picture, enabling you to think things through?
8. Write your behavior—what were your actions in the situation?
9. Give yourself a letter grade for how you behaved. If you were able to recognize your physical cues, calm yourself, act with integrity and without violence, give yourself an A!

Although you are only required to do one journal entry per week, the more you practice this exercise, the better you will get at it.

JOURNAL HOMEWORK Name: Date turned in:

(See binder for instructions)

Date & Time of Day	Describe Situation... ... What Happened?	Intensity: 1-10	Physical Cues	Emotions (other than anger)	Inflammatory Self-Talk	Calming Self-Talk	My Behaviors	Grade (A–B)

(a)

JOURNAL HOMEWORK (sample) Name: Mary Hartwell Date turned in: 2-6-09

(See binder for instructions)

Date & Time of Day	Describe Situation... ... What Happened?	Intensity: 1-10	Physical Cues	Emotions (other than anger)	Inflammatory Self-Talk	Calming Self-Talk	My Behaviors	Grade (A-F)
1-10-09 early morning	My son, Matt, woke me up early to say he had a soccer game...I wanted to sleep in. I thought his game was this afternoon.	3	faster heartbeat	Annoyed, Disappointed, Rushed	I never get to sleep in! His dad should pitch in more. Poor me!	This is important to him. I'm glad he feels responsible to his team. I'll take a nap later.	I thanked him for waking me & took him to the game.	A
1-15-09 afternoon	I was driving to an interview for a job I really want and need... when my car engine started smoking and caught on fire.	10	Racing Heart, Tense all over, Faint, shaky	Overwhelmed, Panicky, Scared, Helpless, Doomed, Powerless.	I should've taken the bus or had a friend drive me. How am I ever going to make it in life???	It's only a car. I am safe, OK. Freaking out isn't going to fix the car or get me to the interview.	I prayed. A Cop pulled up, I told her about probation & interview – she drove me to it!	A
1-23-09 Evening	My fiancé called to cancel our date for tonight because he's sick. We were going to go to dinner and a new movie I really wanted to see.	6	Tense jaw, Tight throat, Hotness all over.	Disappointed, Suspicious, Unimportant, Let down.	I wonder how sick he really is! He just didn't want to see my movie! If it were his turn to choose, he'd go anyway!	I can take him at his word. The flu has been going around. He's more important to me than this movie. I'll survive.	I said I'll take a rain check, does he need me to keep him company? We had a nice evening.	A
1-31-09 afternoon	My ex-husband called to say he was bringing the kids back an hour late because of traffic. I had plans to take them to a BBQ at my friend's.	7	Tension all over, Stomach In knots.	Suspicious, Annoyed, Powerless, Put out.	I can't count on him for anything! He'll be late to his own funeral! Just one of many reasons I divorced him!	It's not always about me. I'm glad the kids are OK and that he called. I will use this extra time to calm down so I can have fun at the BBQ.	I called my friends to say we'd be late. I sat down with my feet up and relaxed.	A

(b)

Figure 10.2a,b Example of journal homework.

Handout: Emotions Inventory

Recognizing and defining our emotions helps us to understand and better express ourselves.

This list of words can help you become more familiar with the language of emotions. When you are not sure how to describe your emotions, read through the list, asking yourself which words most accurately convey how you are feeling.

Positive Emotions			
Happy	Hopeful	Grateful	Comfortable
Content	Giddy	Joyful	Glad
Pleased	Peaceful	Loving	Wonderful
Proud	Loved	Helpful	Valued
Excited	Important	Competent	Free
Confident	Relieved	Amused	Amorous
Delighted	Honorable	Smart	Secure
Safe	Desirable	Curious	Eager
Encouraged	Affirmed	Validated	Comforted
Trusted	Respected	Intimate	Optimistic
Greedy	Honored	Determined	Enlightened

Negative Emotions			
Hurt	Worried	Depressed	Guilty
Sad	Nervous	Ashamed	Confused
Offended	Embarrassed	Humiliated	Afraid
Betrayed	Weak	Cheated	Abandoned
Frustrated	Hopeless	Disgusted	Insecure
Spiteful	Vengeful	Anxious	Inadequate
Jealous	Disappointed	Shy	Isolated
Rejected	Ignored	Insulted	Out of control
Lonely	Aggravated	Challenged	Empty
Vulnerable	Uncomfortable	Ambivalent	Bored
Shocked	Deceitful	Cautious	Annoyed
Used	Afraid	Aggravated	Blamed
Unworthy	Left out	Manipulated	Skeptical
Threatened	Trapped	Violated	Bitter
Uneasy	Sorry	Thwarted	Downhearted
Dejected	Irritable	Resentful	Intimidated
Invalidated	Patronized	Pressured	Hassled
Unglued	Provoked	Overpowered	Animosity
Defensive	Upset	Horrified	Quarrelsome
	Gullible	Troubled	

Handout: Self-Talk: Inflammatory or Calming

Each of us, as we go through day-to-day life, makes interpretations of the things that happen to us. We tell ourselves what these experiences mean about us and those around us. Simply put, this is our self-talk.

What we tell ourselves can determine how we feel—in some pretty amazing and powerful ways—and whether we are likely to take things personally or easily let them go. If we tend to interpret situations in negative ways, we are more likely to feel bad—angry, resentful, or picked on. This can then make it easier to tell ourselves that we are justified in retaliating with violence. Conversely, when we tell ourselves positive interpretations of situations, we are more likely to come away feeling better, calmer, happier with the world around us—and more able to behave nonviolently.

Inflammatory Self-Talk	Calming Self-Talk
If he forgets my birthday, he doesn't love me.	I feel hurt when he forgets my birthday, but he does other things that show me he loves me.
Who does that guy think he is? Cutting me off on the freeway! How rude!	I don't have to take this personally. He may be distracted or have an emergency.
I can't believe my son violated curfew! He's always pushing the limits with me. I have to teach him a lesson!	I'm glad he is all right—that's what's most important. In the morning I can talk calmly with him and find out what happened.
This always happens to me—every red light, and now I'm stuck behind an accident.	I can't control the lights. I'm grateful that I am safe. I can relax and pray for the people in the accident.
He *always* has to win every argument. Jerk! He just wants to show how he's smarter than I am!	He does have strong opinions, but so do I. I can express myself clearly and respectfully. I don't have to change my mind—or his.
My toddler spilled milk on the floor for the third time this week. I think I'm going to lose it!	He's just a little guy—he's still learning. I don't want to scare him. This, too, shall pass. I can stay calm and clean it up, or give him a towel and have him help me clean it up.
He's trying to start a fight to make me act crazy! He wants to get me arrested!	I don't have to get into a fight and I don't have to choose violence.
He's never going to ask me out again. I just know it! Poor me!	I can't read his mind or predict the future. I'll be OK. I can take care of myself.
My daughter always expects me to help with her homework! Whine, whine!	Learning to read is hard. What a nice mom I am to help her!
My boyfriend is talking to a woman at a party. What a flirt! I should go over and set him straight!	I feel left out, but I don't need to make assumptions. Maybe she's the new boss he was telling me about.
If he won't listen to me, I'll throw the remote at him!	Violence isn't going to bring us closer. I can be patient.

Handout: Making Motion Pictures

Sometimes, when we see something, we start to create a story in our mind to explain what we are seeing. This can be entertaining, innocuous, and pass the time—like when watching people at a ball game or crowded amusement park. (For example: The balding man has brought his son and grandson to cheer his lifelong favorite team to victory.... The young couple is on their honeymoon.... The harried parents are trying to persuade their children it is naptime, but the parents are the ones who need the nap!)

Other times, we see something involving our partner. We create a storyline before we know what the truth is and act as if our storyline is the actual truth.

This is called making motion pictures in your head.

Handout: Examples of Calming Self-Talk

- How he behaves reflects on him, not me.
- I don't have to change him—only focus on myself.
- I can stay calm in this situation.
- I don't have to take this personally.
- Rome wasn't built in a day. I can be patient.
- Will I care about this in a day, a week, a year?
- I can acknowledge my feelings, then choose my behavior.
- This, too, shall pass.
- I am powerless over these circumstances. I can let go.
- I made a mistake. I am human. I can learn from this.
- Wisdom is like a pearl: it is built a layer at a time.
- His opinion of me is none of my business. It's his.
- I am in charge of my feelings. No one *makes* me feel any particular way.
- I can't control the direction of the wind, but I can adjust my sails.
- I can have compassion here—for myself, for others.
- I am worthy—simply because I am human, a child of God.
- This situation could be a test. I trust my coping skills. I will be able to figure things out. I don't have to decide right now.
- This isn't worth arguing about. I can express my feelings without escalating the tension.
- Nothing says life is fair. I will handle this with grace and integrity.
- I feel hurt. I am responsible for taking care of my pain. I am
- competent to care for myself.
- Violence won't get me what I want. I can protect myself by speaking assertively.
- He is doing the best he can. I am doing the best I can.
- I'll know *what* I need to know *when* I need to know it. I don't have to stress or worry because I don't know today.
- I don't have to be perfect.
- Relax. Breathe slowly: in calmness, out tension.

Section 4 Binder Contents: Relationship Issues

Suggestions to Therapist

Most of the handouts in this section can be discussed as needed or referred to as women share in group about situations to which the handouts would apply. Additional questions to generate reflection and discussion are as follows:

- Have you ever known a drama queen? She seems like a magnet for upheaval in her life: If there is not a current crisis, she makes one happen. Why do you think some women seem to want to stay "in the drama"? What would have to happen in order for her to change?
- Does relationship violence ever make things better? In the short term? Long run?
- What makes a healthy relationship? (Have the group generate a list and choose the five most important qualities, describing reasoning.)
- What is trust? How can you tell that you have it in your relationship?
- What is respect? How can you tell that you have it your relationship? (Note distinction between treating someone respectfully and respecting him/her.)
- What is intimacy? What is the difference between sex and intimacy? How do you know you have emotional intimacy in your relationship? (Women often confuse sex with intimacy, so this distinction needs to be addressed. This is also a good time to talk about boundaries.)
- In dating, when do you think is the right time to bring up sex? Birth control? Sexually transmitted diseases? (These are good topics to role-play.)
- Have you ever been worried that you would lose a boyfriend if you did not agree to have sex with him? Have you ever said no to any sexual activity? Was it difficult to say? How did it work out? How did this affect your feelings about yourself? The relationship?

Communication Skills

Assertiveness, empathy, coping with criticism, conflict resolution, and healthy communication skills are most effectively taught through role-play. A basic format for expressing oneself clearly and assertively without blame is through "I" messages:

When you (describe behavior) …
    I feel (use feeling words) …
    and I want you to (describe different behavior).

Women (and men) often have difficulty taking ownership of their feelings, especially when upset. When she uses an "I" message, a woman is communicating that she owns her feelings and is responsible for her them. This is in contrast to "you" messages, which blame the other person for her feelings—and ultimately give him power over her.

In addition to suggestions generated by group members, the following are situations that can be role-played. Have several women try out each part.

Role-Plays
- Man comes home from work and did not call to say he would be late.
- Man spent paycheck on video games and booze, so there is not enough money for rent, utilities, and food.
- Man seems suddenly uninterested in sex and rebuffs her overtures.
- When woman wants to talk about their relationship, man walks out.
- Man wants to watch porn, wants her to join him in watching, but she feels uncomfortable.
- Man complains about woman's cooking—"not like mom's."
- Man asks woman why she is having seconds of dessert—Isn't she on a diet?
- Man has custody, says woman cannot see their children unless she has sex with him.
- Man does not get kids to do homework or to bed on time when woman goes out for evening with girlfriends.

Debriefing
In debriefing the actors, ask what their experiences were like. If they were trying to create an argument, did the other person make it difficult? What strategies worked well? When were there examples of assertiveness? Respect for boundaries? "I" messages? Was this difficult to do? Why or why not?

What about the partner: What was he thinking, feeling? Did he think you understood him? How would he describe you and your behavior at that moment? Did you feel understood? What might you have done to make yourself better understood?

Handout: Jealousy

Definition: Fearful of loss of position or affection; resentful in rivalry; envious. Possessively watchful; vigilant (*Webster's Dictionary*).

Motive for jealousy: To protect against deep pain of loss or fear of rejection or abandonment.

Characteristics of people who are vulnerable to jealousy?

- Low self-esteem
- Trauma or loss early in life
- History of physical, psychological, or sexual abuse

Why do people become jealous?

- Their self-worth is tied to how other people respond to them.
- The jealous person is dependent on a partner for something only she (or he) can provide for herself.

> Jealousy is a form of control because of your inability to trust, say no, or set limits.

- How do you know when you are jealous?
- What can you do to resolve your feelings of jealousy, that is nonviolent and respectful?

Suggestions to Therapist: Meaningful Apologies

- **Ask:** Can you think of the last time you apologized or received an apology? Did it repair the relationship? What made the apology meaningful?
- Brainstorm ideas about components of a meaningful apology and write them on the board. Review the binder handout and have group process thoughts about their own experiences.
- **Ask:** What is it like to receive an apology that is heartfelt? One that is empty?

Handout: A Meaningful Apology

How many times have you heard someone say: "Well ... sor-*ry!*" If you are the one who has been hurt and the offense has happened time and again, this "sorry" can feel pretty empty.

Meaningful apologies are heartfelt and sincere. They convey to the injured not only remorse but also the desire and intention to change.

Think about the last time you apologized or received an apology. Did it include these four important components:

1. Acknowledging that someone was hurt
2. Taking full responsibility for his or her own part
3. Demonstrating compassion or empathy for the hurt person
4. Offering to make up for the hurt (in a way that has meaning to the injured person)

The ultimate goal of a meaningful apology is to repair and restore a broken relationship, but this is not guaranteed. The other person retains the right to make his or her own decision about forgiveness. Apologizing and forgiveness are separate issues.

Suggestions to Therapist: Forgiveness

- **Ask:** Think about a time that you were forgiven. What was the offense? Who forgave you? How? What was the outcome of the act of forgiveness?
- **Ask:** Think about a time that you forgave someone for an offense to you. What did this person do? When and how did you forgive? What happened to your anger after you forgave?
- **Ask:** Are there some violations that are so egregious that they cannot be forgiven? What are those? What seems impossible about forgiving them? Is acceptance a possible alternative?

Forgiveness can be difficult and controversial. No one can dictate to another that she *must* forgive—it is the right of the injured to make that choice. Pressuring someone to forgive when she is not ready is a serious boundary violation that only deepens the original wound.

Handout: Forgiveness

The very nature of human relationships guarantees that we will have times when we feel hurt and when we hurt those we most love. Forgiveness is challenging, difficult, and *necessary*. It means letting go of the right to resentments.

Forgiveness *is not*:

- Forgetting what happened
- Excusing a person for what he or she did
- Deserved

Forgiveness *is*:

- Acknowledging your emotions
- Deciding to forgive
- Surrendering the right to get even
- Finding redemptive meaning in the experience

Questions to consider:

- Who does the forgiveness benefit?
- How does it benefit or harm me to forgive—or chose not to?
- Is there a part of me that resists forgiving because to do so would mean I lose power over that person?
- Am I reluctant to give up my position of moral superiority?
- Do I know what I want to hear from the other person?

Consider these thoughts:

- Waiting for someone to repent before we forgive is to surrender our future to the person who wronged us.
- We do our forgiving alone, inside our hearts and minds; what happens to the people we forgive depends on them.
- Forgiving does not require us to reunite with the person who broke our trust.
- To give forgiveness requires nothing but a desire to be free of our resentments. To receive forgiveness requires sorrow for what we did to give someone reason to be resentful.

Wisdom From "The Forgiveness Project—Stories":

- The deeper the wound, the longer the journey.
- We do not forgive because we are supposed to; we forgive when we are ready to be healed.
- Forgiving is not a way to avoid pain but to heal pain.
- When we forgive, we set a prisoner free and discover the prisoner we set free is us.

---

* www.theforgivenessproject.com ("Stories"). Reprinted with permission.

Suggestion to Therapist: Social Intelligence and Empathy

The therapist may review the following information and share it with the group as the "Empathy" handout is discussed.

Author and psychologist Daniel Goleman (2006, p. 251) says that social intelligence is being intelligent about relationships. He says there are two components:

1. **Empathy:** Using your emotional radar to sense what another person is feeling and understand what his intentions are, so you can decide, for example, if you can trust him.
2. **Social skills:** Knowing what to say and how to time things so your interactions with another person are effective and you *both* get what you want or need. Being manipulative—valuing only what works for one person at the expense of the other—is not social intelligence.

Goleman says that our brains are wired for connection with others. The more intimately we are attached, the stronger the brain connection. Our eyes contain nerves that lead directly to a part of the brain that triggers empathy—the orbitofrontal cortex (OFC). The OFC stimulates nearby cells called mirror neurons. These neurons allow us to intuit each other's emotions, sense and coordinate our facial expressions, and play a key role in developing rapport. (Sounds like what happens in good therapy!)

Can I improve my social intelligence? Yes. Try the following:

1. Strengthen your brain for empathy by consciously and repeatedly paying more attention to others. Empathy is strongest when we fully focus on someone else; self-absorption kills empathy.
2. Help a child learn how to calm down by modeling healthy behavior; for instance, refrain from getting angry in reaction to the child's anger. This strengthens the part of the brain involved in resilience—the ability to recover from upset.
3. Have relationships that repair bad things that happened to you in the past. These can rewire the neural scripts from childhood (e.g., therapy, partner and friends who are empathic, nurturing).
4. Master a relaxation technique such as deep, slow breathing, yoga, or meditation. Practice it when you are calm so you can use it when you are very upset.

Handout: Empathy

Empathy is the ability to put yourself in someone else's shoes, to feel what they are feeling from their perspective. It is not sympathy—looking down on the other person, feeling pity for him or her. Why is empathy important? It helps us understand each other and feel understood. It helps us feel accepted and cared for. Empathy can be difficult, especially when the topic is emotionally charged for us personally.

These are the steps for empathy:

1. Listen carefully to the other person.
2. Imagine what emotions he or she might be feeling.
3. Why do you think he or she might be feeling that way?
4. Check out your perception; ask if you are understanding correctly.

Consider the following. Which responses do you think convey empathy? Why?

1. Your six-year-old daughter comes home from school crying. "I don't have any friends! Nobody likes me! Everybody else in my class but me got invited to Mary's birthday party."
   a. "There'll be other birthday parties. Besides, I thought you didn't like Mary!"
   b. "When I was your age I *never* got invited to parties."
   c. "That's hard when other kids are talking about something that sounds so fun and you aren't a part of it. Are you feeling left out or all alone?"
2. Your friend calls: "I decided I don't need to go to NA meetings anymore. I'm tired of all those depressing, loser stories. I can stay clean on my own."
   a. "Are you sure that's a good idea? Have you talked to your sponsor about it?"
   b. "You sound positive about your decision, and the meetings weren't helping you feel good anymore, right?"
   c. "I'll really miss seeing you there! I always liked hearing your perspective on the things we talk about."
3. Your husband comes home late from work: "My boss is impossible! All he did was yell at us all day long, like none of us could do things right or move fast enough. What a jerk!"
   a. "You sound like you are feeling exhausted. I know you work really hard and are a good employee. Are you feeling unappreciated?"
   b. "Sounds like a hard day for your whole crew. Is he feeling the heat from the owner of the company?"
   c. "You think your boss is a jerk? Just be glad you don't have mine!"

Remember: Empathy is simply acknowledging the emotions you sense the other person is having. It does not mean offering an unsolicited opinion. It is not about trying to change his feelings, giving reasons he should not feel the way he does, or trying to make him feel better. It is not about judging. It is not about making yourself feel better in the guise of helping the other person. It is about understanding.

Suggestions to Therapist

The purpose of the handout on boundaries is:

- To educate women about what boundaries are
- To help them recognize when they are succeeding or failing at maintaining their own boundaries
- To help them recognize when someone else is respecting or violating their boundaries or those of their children

The handout "Sex and Intimacy" is included in a discussion of boundaries because this is often an area of women's lives where they have difficulty defining, establishing, and enforcing healthy boundaries for themselves.

A Word About Boundaries: The Poker Analogy

Sometimes during arguments, women will tell former partners of their plans, thinking that the information will make him change his mind or behave differently. They waste energy arguing. For example, when Miriam and Joe argue, he clenches his fists, screams, calls her names, and throws things at her. She is on probation and is afraid to retaliate like she used to, so she tells him that he better stop because next time she is going to call the police.

In cases like these, the poker analogy may be helpful. In poker, if you want to win, you do not let your opponents know what is in your hand and you do not give clues. You keep your cards close to your chest and play your hand. Translated to Miriam and Joe's situation, this means that Miriam does not tell Joe her plans—he does not need to know ahead of time; she simply carries them out—she calls the police.

It should be pointed out that this analogy is not meant to recommend that arguments or relationships be viewed as games. Poker can provide a powerful visual metaphor for when a woman needs to disengage from a destructive, enmeshed battle—and think.

Handout: Boundaries

Good fences make good neighbors.

Robert Frost

The same could be said of boundaries and healthy relationships.

Good boundaries are the limits that define who we are, separate from one another. They define how we are in relationship to others and ourselves. They bring order to our lives. They protect us by helping us to know what is safe and appropriate and what is not.

Boundaries can be

- Physical (our skin, the space that our body takes up, the invisible space we need between us and others)
- Emotional (our feelings, reactions, perceptions, values, concerns, goals)
- Spiritual (our knowledge and experience of what we believe spiritually)
- Sexual (our limits on what is safe and appropriate behavior from and with others)
- Relational (our limits of what is appropriate interaction with others)

The process of boundary development begins early in life as we each form a self-concept that is separate, individual, and unique from our parents and other family members.

A boundary violation occurs when someone (whether intentional or not) crosses the physical, emotional, spiritual, sexual, or relational limits of another person. It does not matter if the violator has good intentions; it is still a boundary violation because it causes harm. A violation says that what I believe, who I am, what I feel and want does not matter.

Establishing good boundaries begins with self-awareness. Ask yourself:

- How do I feel?
- Am I angry? Guilty? Resentful? Frightened?
- Do I feel used? Violated? Isolated? Like a child?
- Is someone else's behavior toward me OK? Am I comfortable with this?
- What do I really want? What is important to me?
- Are my boundaries healthy? Are they too rigid, keeping me apart when I want to feel connected? Are they too flexible, making me vulnerable to abuse or manipulation?

We each have the right to define our own boundaries, have ours respected, and respect those of others. Sometimes, though, people close to us may protest our newly defined sense of ourselves. If this happens, listen to the objection (as long as it is stated respectfully), restate the boundary, and stick with it. If you want to reconsider or change the boundary, think about it away from the person who is trying to change your mind.

Handout: Sex and Intimacy

Sex and intimacy are two very different things. Each can be experienced separately in relationships, or they can be experienced at the same time. Sex alone is only sex, but with intimacy, it can be amazing! These questions are for your own reflection. You will not be asked to share answers in group unless you feel comfortable doing so.

- How did you find out about sex? What attitude was conveyed about sex in your family of origin? How did you find out about masturbation, menstruation, pregnancy, birth control, etc.? How has this affected you?

- When was your first sexual experience? Did you see yourself as a willing participant, or did you feel pressured, confused, forced, humiliated, or intimidated? If you were forced, did you tell anyone? What was their response? How has this affected you and subsequent experiences and relationships?

- As an adult, what function does sex have in your life and your partnership? Do you and your partner talk about your sexual relationship—when you are *not* being sexual?

- Which is more important to you—sex or intimacy? Why?

- Who makes most of the decisions about sex, birth control, pregnancy— you or your partner? Why do you think that is?

- How do you decide when to have sex in a relationship? When is "too soon"?

- If you are in a committed relationship, is flirting with others OK? Why or why not?

- Is it OK to cheat sexually on your partner? Have you ever cheated? Has your partner? Why do you think this happened? What was the effect on each of you, on the relationship?

Suggestions to Therapist

The next four handouts are:

- "Coping With Criticism"
- "Understanding Assertiveness"
- "Constructive Conflict and Problem Solving"
- "The Cycle of Violence"

These are self-explanatory and can be reviewed and discussed at any point during the group. It is always a good idea to encourage women to read their binders between group meetings. Often, they will share in group that they were having a hard time with a particular situation, decided to read the binder, and found helpful information for that situation.

Handout: Coping with Criticism

All of us experience criticism sometime in life. When it comes from some-one whose opinions matter most to us, we can feel like we have been deeply wounded at our core. Learning to cope with criticism can help us feel better about ourselves, establish and maintain healthy interpersonal boundaries, and improve our relationships. Consider these suggestions:

- Whether or not you take offense at someone's criticism of you is a *choice*. The decision is up to you.
- Accept criticism nondefensively.
- View criticism as constructive feedback intended to help you be a better person.
- Ask for more information.
- Remind yourself that you do not have to be perfect. It is OK to make mistakes and acknowledge them.
- Is there a part of the criticism that is true? Agreeing with the part that is true can go a long way in diffusing an argument. You do not have to agree with the part that is untrue.
- You may decide that the criticism is unjustified. It is OK to disagree. You can still stay in control of your behaviors and decisions.
- Sometimes criticism is delivered in a manner that is aggressive or hostile. It is OK to set limits with the other person. "I want to hear what you have to say, but I can't while you are calling me names."
- Criticism may catch you by surprise. You may feel overwhelmed, hurt, or confused. It is OK to not respond in the moment and take a time-out. "I'll have to think more about that and get back to you."
- If the criticism is justified, apologize, acknowledge the other person's feelings, and make a commitment to change.

No one can make you feel inferior without your consent. <div align="right">Eleanor Roosevelt</div>

Using the above suggestions, how could you respond to these situations:

- Your husband says: "I work hard all day and come home to a pig sty! Don't you do anything but watch TV when I'm at work?"
- After telling your five-year-old daughter it is time to clean up and go to bed, she yells: "You're the meanest mommy in the world! I hate you! I'm never inviting you to my birthday party!"
- Your father says: "When are you going to leave that loser boyfriend of yours? Didn't I raise you to expect better than that?"

Handout: Understanding Assertiveness

When you are assertive, you are confident in yourself. You know what you feel, think, and want; you are able to state these honestly, clearly, and respectfully. You also know what you do not want and are able to directly refuse it. Generally, men's assertiveness is accepted more in our society than women's, and often women confuse assertiveness with aggressiveness. Consider the four different styles of behavior below.

Assertive

You are appropriately direct and honest. You express your feelings, thoughts, and needs while being empathic and respectful toward the other person. You can disagree without being disrespectful. Your express your own thoughts and feelings without being judgmental or blaming. You accept full responsibility for yourself and your behavior.

Aggressive

You may confuse this with assertiveness, which it is not. If you are being aggressive, you might be honest and direct, but inappropriately so. When you express yourself, you come across as righteous, superior, entitled, controlling, blaming, attacking, hostile, and sometimes violent. You are more interested in getting your own way or expressing your opinion than being respectful of the other person.

Passive

Rather than speaking up about your own thoughts, feelings, needs, and desires, you allow others to make decisions for you and about you. You may adopt the position of martyr, telling yourself you are doing the noble thing by making sacrifices. In reality, this style of behavior is emotionally dishonest and insecure. Passive people tend to apologize or blame others, rather than expressing themselves honestly, directly, and respectfully.

Passive–Aggressive

Rather than directly asking for what you want, you are emotionally dishonest and express your thoughts, feelings, and needs covertly, indirectly. Your words may say one thing and your behavior the opposite. This can cause great confusion in others because you do not take responsibility for your behavior.

Handout: Constructive Conflict and Problem Solving

All couples have conflicts. Psychologist John Gottman, PhD, (1994) of University of Washington, has researched couples for over 30 years. He has found that couple conflicts fall in one of two categories: perpetual problems and solvable problems.

Gottman says that 69% of the conflicts couples have are about perpetual problems—those based on differences in personality and lifestyle (he is chronically messy and she is a neat freak; she is always late and he likes to be early; he wants sex every day and she wants it twice a week). Solvable problems are situational and time; limited (he wants her to go bowling and she wants a night out with girlfriends, she wants him to help more with child care and he says that when he tries, the baby cries).

The solution for both types of problems is the same: communicating basic acceptance of your partner's personality. To *get* understanding you have to *give* understanding. To influence your partner, you have to accept influence.

In stable relationships, couples find ways to cope effectively with the perpetual problems and focus on solving the solvable problems. Gottman recommends five steps for resolving conflict, whether over perpetual or solvable problems:

1. Soften your start-up when addressing a complaint.
2. Learn to make and receive repair attempts.
3. Soothe yourself and each other.
4. Compromise.
5. Be tolerant of each other's faults.

Ask yourself:

What do I want from my partner?
Do I want him to make me feel better?
Do I want him to understand me better?
Do I understand his side? Have I validated his thoughts and feelings?
Do I want him to do something for me? If he does, will this help me feel more capable and compassionate?

Guidelines for respectful communication and negotiation about conflicts:

- Be respectful. No yelling, no threatening or violent behavior, no name calling.
- Each person's opinion and feelings are valid.
- Stay focused on the issue on the table.
- Define the problem. Who is affected and how?
- What are the immediate and long-term goals?
- What are possible solutions? Is there one that will meet both partners' needs?

Handout: The Cycle of Violence

In her book *The Battered Woman Syndrome*, Lenore Walker (1984) says that domestic violence follows a three-phase cycle. One phase leads to the next, each fueled by denial to keep that keeps the cycle going.

Tension-Building Phase

- He is moody, irritable, critical, calls her names, belittles her, isolates her, threatens.
- She tries to calm him by being nurturing, compliant, agreeable.
- She accepts his abusive behavior in order to prevent escalation.
- He thinks he's the victim and blames her, believes he is entitled to a certain response from her.
- If she cries or objects, he tells her to toughen up, that she is too sensitive.
- They have a silent agreement: He thinks, "She's bad"; she thinks, "I guess I am."
- The tension becomes unbearable.

Acute Battering or Explosion Phase

- He wants to teach her a lesson.
- He is violent to her: hitting, beating, choking, raping, shoving, punching, and so forth.
- He does not care what happens or the consequences, and blames her.
- She tries to wait out the storm rather than fighting back, protecting herself however she can.
- Neighbors, children, or friends may call police.
- After the violence: shock, denial, disbelief—and relief that it is over.
- Both try to rationalize, make excuses.
- Women who go to the emergency room often return to their partners.

Contrition Phase

- He begs forgiveness, promises to never do it again, promises to go to church, go to AA, do whatever she wants.
- He gives her flowers, candy, gifts, and so forth.
- He reminds her of how much he needs her.
- She wants to believe him, feels confused.
- She sees how wonderful he can be, reinforcing her hope that violence will stop.
- She minimizes her injuries, tells herself, "It could have been worse."
- She agrees to reconcile, stops any legal proceedings, sets up counseling appointment for him.
- Victimization of the woman becomes complete.
- A period of calm is welcomed by both of them.
- Each is dependent on the other; bonding occurs.
- The stage is set to return to the tension-building phase. The cycle continues.

Section 5 Binder Contents: Family of Origin

Suggestions to Therapist

Addressing family of origin issues is the most powerful, transforming experience in this program. It is during this exercise that group members are most emotionally vulnerable, self-disclosing, and compassionate—for themselves and for the others in the group.

Sharing family of origin, attachment style, and narrative is designed to provide a reparative experience—through attunement provided by the therapist and the rest of the group, empathy, and healing of attachment trauma. The individual client who is sharing and the group as a whole dictate the pace at which information is shared and processed. The therapist must be vigilant to notice when it is time to pursue and when it is time to back off.

The family of origin part of the program is addressed after a woman has been attending group for a while, has begun to feel comfortable in group, and is able to self-disclose. Because only one woman shares her family of origin per week, it can take a few months for the whole group to complete this. The binder information about family of origin, attachment, and narratives can be addressed and discussed for a couple of weeks before the first woman shares her story.

Beginning with the most senior group member allows newer ones to best benefit from her modeling. It is important that a woman know ahead of time which group meeting she will be sharing her family of origin.

Preparing the Group for Family of Origin

The therapist may say: In this program, we think that understanding your family of origin—your childhood experiences—is essential. It helps you to answer two questions: How did my childhood experiences shape me to be the woman I am today? What is the connection between my past and my ending up in this program? If you can answer these questions for yourself, you are empowered to make choices from here on out about the type of woman you want to be and how you want to live your life. Learning from history allows us to not repeat it.

Then, over a couple of weeks, the therapist can have the group read through the handouts entitled "Family of Origin," "Attunement and

Attachment," "Four Attachment Styles," and "Coherent Narrative." These contain a lot of information that can be difficult to absorb, so it can be helpful to review key concepts periodically (i.e., ask: Why is family of origin important? What do you remember about attachment?).

Ask each woman to be thinking about what she wants to share with the group when it is her turn.

The therapist may say: For all of us, our family of origin is the template by which we understand ourselves and relationships. Before we have conscious memory, we learn what to expect from those who take care of us, and what we must do to get our basic needs met.

We learn our *family rules*. Each family has them. They are the spoken and unspoken rules that dictate how we should or should not behave in any particular situation. Spoken rules may include things such as mealtimes, bedtimes, curfews, and chores. Unspoken rules are those that everyone is aware of but never mentions: mom's affair, dad's drinking, grandpa molesting several grandkids, the baby brother who died from SIDS.

Family rules also govern how the family interacts with each other. How are emotions expressed—especially love and anger? Are some emotions or behaviors OK for some, such as parents, but not for others, such as children? Are the rules realistic, or humanly possible? What gets talked about and what gets swept under the carpet, as if it doesn't exist? If something important does not get talked about, how does that impact a child's ability to trust, be comforted and reassured, feel safe? What are the rules about sharing information? Are the rules flexible enough?

In examining family rules, it is also important to consider *roles* within the family. Do the adults take care of the children, or vice versa? When there is conflict, how does each of the children respond (e.g., becoming invisible, acting out, being a clown and making jokes, getting in the middle of the parents to negotiate a truce, trying harder to be more perfect so parents won't be unhappy)?

Rarely does anyone come from a perfect childhood. In fact, most people have something they wish was different about their own childhood. Sometimes, women feel guilty for talking about their families. This exercise is not about blaming your family or finding fault. It is about helping you to have *perspective and self-awareness*, to be able to better understand yourself and *create meaning* out of your family of origin experiences.

Handout: Family of Origin

For each of us, our family of origin is the template for our understanding of ourselves and relationships. It is where we learn what mothers are like, what fathers are like, how mothers and fathers interact with each other, how adults interact with children, how emotions are expressed, how problems are resolved. For each of us, it is our frame of reference, what feels normal.

As you plan what you choose to share in group about your family of origin, consider the following questions. Remember, the goal is not to blame, but rather to consider how *you* were affected by what you experienced, and how this has informed your beliefs about yourself and relationships.

- What was my relationship with my mother like?
  What did I learn about women and men from my mother?
  What was missing from my relationship with my mother?
  How did this affect who I became and the way I feel about myself today?
- What was my relationship with my father like?
  What did I learn about women and men from my father?
  What was missing from my relationship with my father?
  How did this affect who I became and the way I feel about myself today?
- What did I learn about love from the way my mother and father treated each other? From how they treated me?
  What does "close relationship" mean to me?
- How did my parents settle their differences? Was there domestic violence? Who was violent? What happened? Where was I? How did I feel? How did this affect me?
- Did either of my parents abuse alcohol or drugs? How did this affect their ability to parent me?
- How was I punished as a child?
- Was I abused—physically, emotionally, sexually? What was the relationship of the abuser to me? Did I tell either of my parents? How do I think this affected me?
- What feelings were most dominant or familiar to me as I was growing up?
- If my feelings were hurt, if I was upset or angry, how did I deal with it?

Who helped me and how?

As you reflect on what you will share with the group about your childhood experiences, also come prepared to share what you see as your coherent narrative and your attachment style.

Suggestions to Therapist: Attachment Style

(See Chapter 2 for discussion of Mary Ainsworth's research on attachment.) Mary Ainsworth learned about attachment styles by studying toddlers and their mothers. She instructed the mother to leave the child in a room with some toys and a stranger, and then observed and recorded the child's and mother's responses as the mother left and then returned. (Review "Attunement and Attachment" and "Four Attachment Styles" handouts.)

Attachment is something that happens from the time we are born. It is essential to our survival because it is where we learn how to be close, intimate, how to trust, and how to be autonomous, independent. It is the process through which we learn to self-soothe. When we have a consistent, safe, responsive adult, we feel protected in times of distress (safe harbor) and yet freed to venture out and explore the world, because we have someone to lean on (secure base). We feel safe and supported. This group is designed to provide each of you a safe harbor and a secure base.

When a caregiver is inconsistent, rejecting, shaming, or abusive, a child learns to make compromises to avoid losing what little attachment she may have. She chronically searches for a secure base. She feels dependent and isolated. The patterns enacted through her childhood attachments are likely to be the same ones she will enact in adulthood.

Handout: Attunement and Attachment

Our earliest experiences of attunement happen when we are infants. When we cry, our mother (or other caregiver) interprets the meaning of the cries—hunger, poopy diaper, lonely, bored, sick, tired, and so forth. When mom gets it right and responds to our need, we feel connected, validated, safe, satisfied; we experience attunement. When she does not respond or consistently misinterprets our needs, we experience abandonment and rage.

Just as a child's needs change as she grows, the expression of attunement valso changes. What remains the same is the child's need for mom to accurately read her.

A toddler needs to feel safe to explore the world and safe to return to mom for reassurance. Mom looks for signals from her child to know *when* she needs to "launch" (i.e., crawl and play with toys) and when she needs to return and connect (i.e., be held). The mother provides her child with a secure base to leave and explore the world, and a safe harbor to return to when the world seems stormy. (Figure 10.3)

This process of reading, letting go, and welcoming back continues throughout childhood (and for the rest of our lives). As a child grows, she experiences that she is a human being separate from others and with her own unique, individual identity. She experiences that she is comforted in times of distress and has someone to lean on when we needs to move forward.

The quality of these experiences will determine her capacity for trust, autonomy, and intimacy, how she will see herself, and what she will expect from her important relationships in life—her attachment relationships.

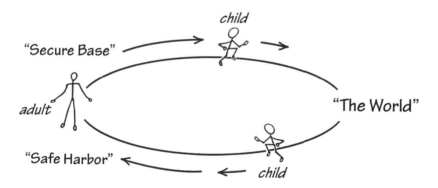

Attunement → Secure Attachment

Figure 10.3   From attunement to secure attachment.

Handout: Four Attachment Styles

Secure Attachment in Childhood

Child:

Protests mother's departure, seeks comfort and calms quickly on mother's return

Accepts reassurance and then returns to exploration (playing with toys)

Mother:

Consistently responsive and accurate in reading child's unspoken emotional cues

Picks up child and soothes her when distressed, puts her down when she wants to explore

Confident in her parenting, available, and responsive

Shows empathy and an ability to talk about emotions

Leads to Secure/Autonomous Adult

- Most likely to describe themselves and partners in a positive light
- Value attachment-related experiences
- Have an accurate understanding of important relationships in their lives
- Show compassion for others
- Able to speak coherently about how past has influenced present feelings and relationships
- Comfortable with emotional intimacy and do not often worry about being abandoned

Insecure/Avoidant Attachment in Childhood

Child:

Shows no outward signs of distress at mother's departure, avoids eye contact on return by appearing to be busy with toys, wards off any advances the mother makes

Mother:

Appears unaware of her child's distress

Gruff when handling her child

Avoids close body contact or rebuffs the child's bids for comfort

Leads to Insecure/Dismissive Adult

- Experience close relationships as too much trouble
- Appear independent to a fault, as if they do not need anyone
- Tend to deny that childhood attachment experiences had influence on present behavior
- Deal with rejection by distancing themselves and suppressing feelings
- Tend to dissociate sexual from emotional commitment
- Uncomfortable with emotional self-disclosure

Insecure/Ambivalent Attachment in Childhood

Child:

Very distressed at the mother's departure

Anxious and angry at her return, clingy and unable to let go and explore

Mother:

Significantly less attuned to her child's emotional states and unspoken needs

Inconsistently responsive

More likely to ignore her child when distressed and to intrude when the child is happily playing

Leads to Insecure/Preoccupied or Ambivalent Adult

- Clingy, fall in love too easily
- Reveal themselves too quickly and too early in relationships
- Can be excessively jealous and possessive
- Often view partners as fickle and undependable
- Worry that partners do not really love them or will leave

Insecure/Disorganized Attachment in Childhood

Child:

Behavior is often extreme

Behavior vacillates between avoidance and ambivalence on mother's departure and return

No strategy for managing anxiety

Mother:

Like her child, shows great distress when her child is distressed

Appears to have no consistent strategy for responding to her child

No awareness of her role in her child's difficulties

Often has childhood history of abuse or suffered a profound early loss, e.g., death of parent

Leads to Insecure/Unresolved or Disorganized/Fearful Adult

- Fear both intimacy and abandonment
- Tend to be overly demanding and angry
- Hypersensitive to rejection in their adult intimate relationships

Suggestions to Therapist: Narratives

Each of us has a life narrative; we just may not recognize it. A life narrative is a simple statement that summarizes what we have come to believe about ourselves and what we can expect from life, from relationships. The value in putting your narrative into words—making it "coherent"—is that you can then take a step back and decide if that is what you want to continue to tell yourself—or if you want to revise your narrative.

Handout: Coherent Narrative

A narrative is an internal working model that reflects our predominant view of ourselves and the world. It influences, determines, and guides our decisions in whom we choose as intimate partners.

Having a coherent narrative means understanding how past experiences are linked to present ways of perceiving ourselves and others, and how these perceptions affect our behavior.

It is a fundamental aspect of insight and self-awareness. When partners have an understanding of how their pasts have affected them, they are less likely to repeat dysfunctional interactions from their families of origin in their present relationships.

Being able to recognize and define your narrative provides the path to a new narrative.

What did you come to believe about yourself, and what you could expect from close relationships? What has been your narrative?

Suggestions to Therapist

The group experience when a woman shares her family of origin:

The therapist may say: In many ways, this group works like a family—a healthy family. What happens in a healthy family? When a member is sharing personal, sensitive information and feelings, the rest of the family listens attentively and respectfully. They *pay really good attention.* They ask her questions that help her deepen her understanding of herself, and they show that they care about her. They treat her in a way that demonstrates profound concern and respect. They respond to her with their own authentic feelings and they try to be helpful to her.

Sharing about your family of origin can mean talking about things you have never talked about before. That takes a lot of courage, especially when you are feeling vulnerable. So, what happens in a healthy family? They do not simply hear the words; they say something that conveys that they have heard and care. They demonstrate empathy and compassion.

When (Mary) has told us what she wants to share about herself, you will be able to ask her questions to better understand her. At the very end, we will go around the room with each group member responding individually to (Mary) about what she has told us.

Also important: Pay attention to a woman's body language affect as she shares. Does she seem emotionally disconnected from the content of her story? Is she flooded with emotions as she recalls her past? If so, it may be necessary to stop her, ask if she is aware, for example, that she is smiling while she is telling about horrific experiences in childhood. The goal is to help her reconnect emotions to content.

Summarized Examples

Renee, in her early 30s, describes a childhood where her family was part of a large, extended family. Many weekends were spent with the adults together, staying up all night drinking, playing music, and sometimes getting into fistfights, while the many cousins ran around the grandparents' farm. She was one of the youngest and described herself as obedient and happy. She felt loved by both parents.

When she was 5, an older male cousin enticed her to go with him to see some newborn kittens in the barn. There, he molested her. She did not really understand what happened. The next day, while mom was nursing a hangover, Renee told her what her cousin had done. Mom got angry with her, told her not to lie, that her cousin would never do such a wicked thing, and besides, she had bigger things to deal with. She tried to tell her dad, but unbeknownst to her, he had had a big argument with her mom the night before. Her parents had decided he must move out because he had been having an affair with her mom's sister. Dad was crying as he packed his things and told her she may never see him again. (She didn't for five years, and then only occasionally.) Renee felt suddenly alone.

Since age 5, when she tried to tell her mom about the molestation, she has never told anyone else—until telling the group.

When she was 15, she married the first boy she had sex with, because he paid attention to her. They had three children right away, and she told herself they were happy. He got laid off his job and started drinking more. When she asked him for money to buy food for the kids, he told her to "go turn some tricks" and laughed. One night he came home drunk and confessed that he had been screwing her girlfriend. She exploded, knocking him out with a fireplace poker.

Attachment style: Insecure—preoccupied or ambivalent.

Narrative: "Even though I try to be good, I can't be good enough. If I want to be loved, I have to take whatever I can get and hold on tight, so he doesn't leave me."

Group response: Some cried. All told her that they believed her story about being molested and were proud of her courage as such a little girl to go and tell her mom. They told her she did not deserve what happened to her and that they felt sad that she had to go through that experience. They told her they felt angry with the cousin who molested her and wished they could have prevented it from happening. They told her they felt honored that she trusted the group enough to tell them. They pointed out her good qualities and told her she is worthy of being loved, treated respectfully, and feeling safe.

Melody, in her late 20s, was taken from her mom by Child Protective Services (CPS) when she was 7, after a police officer found Melody and her younger brother rummaging through trash behind a grocery store looking for food. Mom was addicted to meth and dad was long gone. CPS tried to help mom get clean and sober, but without success.

Melody and her brother went back and forth for five years between mom and foster homes (16 total) until mom relinquished parental rights and a foster family adopted the two children. The family provided food, clothing, and shelter but was demanding, punitive, and shaming—the mom, in particular. Melody was often compared to the family's biological children and told how she did not measure up.

As Melody entered puberty, the adoptive mom called her a slut and predicted she would be pregnant by 13. She did not get pregnant, but she did discover alcohol and drugs. She came home late from a party one night, drunk and stoned. Her adoptive family kicked her out.

Because she was very bright, she was able to pass her high school equivalency exam early. She worked a series of jobs and began a job training program through the local community college. She dropped out. She was a strikingly beautiful young woman who had many boyfriends—most of them drug and sex buddies. These relationships were short-lived—usually ending after she had an angry meltdown over some perceived slight and physically beat up the boyfriend. One of those incidents led to her arrest.

Attachment style: Insecure—disorganized/fearful.

Narrative: "I am fatally flawed, a loser. I will never be loved by anyone. I am helpless to avoid getting hurt again. My future is hopeless."

Group response: Many remarked they never would have guessed she had had such a disruptive, rejecting childhood if she had not revealed the story. Many told her she did not deserve the sad, sad childhood she had had. They reminded her of how she had given them good advice at different times and told her they were grateful to her. They pointed out to her the progress she had already made by staying clean and sober, and suggested that this is a turning point in her life—the bad things are in the past and now she can make her life what she wants. They offered her hope.

Terri, in her mid 30s, began her story by saying she does not like to talk about herself and does not think she has a very interesting story to tell, especially compared to others.

She was an only child raised by a single mother who often left her home alone for days at a time to be with her boyfriend. Sometimes mom left money on the kitchen table and told Terri to take care of herself; other times she forgot. If mom had a fun time with her boyfriend, she came home happy and wanted to tell Terri all about it. If she had fought with her boyfriend, mom would be irritable when she got home and tell Terri to leave her alone.

Terri learned to cook, do laundry, and get herself to and from school. As she put it to the group, she raised herself "without any parental guidance." No one at school suspected that she was usually home alone. She did not have friends over to the house and did not go to other kids' houses.

After she graduated from high school, she enrolled in college. She decided to focus on her career and was surprised when another student expressed interest in dating her. They had a whirlwind affair and she fell in love—or at least that is what she told herself in the moment. Now, she thinks she was just "in lust." They broke up after he had accused her of being cold and closed off. She had a few one-night stands—one that ended up in a fight in front of her apartment building. Neighbors called police when they saw her throw car keys at a man and he fell to the ground clutching his face. The keys hit him hard enough to cut his face and scratch his eye.

Attachment style: Insecure—avoidant/dismissive.

Narrative: "I don't need other people because they can't really be counted on—they all have their own problems. I need to be really careful and not let anyone know what I'm really thinking or feeling—otherwise I'll get hurt or rejected."

Group response: Initially, the group was quiet, like in shock. One by one the women told Terri that when she was home alone, she was the same ages as their own young children, whom they see as innocent, vulnerable. They told her they imagined it must have been very frightening to be alone so much. They added that she must have been an exceptionally brave and capable little girl to teach herself to do so much by herself, but that it was not fair, she did not deserve it, she was the kind of little girl they would be proud to have as their own. She deserved to be loved.

When women share their own family of origin information, they may have difficulty articulating a revised, healthier narrative for themselves. Often the healthier narrative is suggested through the responses of the other women to the one that was shared. The therapist can underscore and tie them together to suggest a new, more hopeful narrative.

Additional questions that can be discussed during this phase of group:

- What can I do to provide a secure base/safe harbor for my children?
- What are the effects of domestic violence on children? How can this be repaired?
- What do you think our culture or the media tell us about girls, attachment, relationships, and violence? How has this affected you and your attitudes about violence?

The following three handouts are

- "Effects of Domestic Violence on Children"
- "Parenting Nonviolently: Teaching Our Children"
- "Co-Parenting With an Ex-Partner"

They provide framework and guidance for answering these questions.

Handout: Effects of Domestic Violence on Children

Common difficulties of children in an abusive family:

- Sleeping problems
- Frequent periods of sadness or crying
- Depression (may look like chronic boredom)
- Anxiety
- School problems
- Difficulty concentrating
- Aggressiveness
- Hyperactivity
- Low self-esteem
- Fearful
- Blunted emotions

A child who grows up in a violent family:

- Learns to use violence in relationships
- Learns to deny fear, because fear equals weakness
- Learns that violence equals love
- Learns to be hypervigilant, on guard
- Learns that people can't be trusted

A child who witnesses domestic violence is

- Ten times more likely to become either an abuser or a victim of abuse
- As an adult, at increased risk of alcoholism, depression, and/or anxiety

---

Seeing or hearing domestic violence *is* child abuse.

Handout: Parenting Nonviolently: Teaching Our Children

No parent is perfect, but child abuse in never the child's fault.

Being a parent is hard work. It means remembering the big picture in each of the little moments. It means remembering our ultimate goal: teaching our children self-control and how to get along so that they can grow to become responsible, caring adults.

This can be especially challenging for parents to remember when we are tired, stressed out, or angry, or when our child is misbehaving, lying, or having a tantrum.

Remember: We teach our children most effectively by example, *how we behave*, rather than by what we *tell* them.

- Be realistic about where your child is developmentally.
- Set appropriate limits. Present options, but not too many.
- Reduce triggers. Is your child hungry, tired, getting sick?
- Don't take your child's words or behavior personally.
- Children, like adults, also have real feelings and need to be able to express them.

Listen to what they are trying to say rather than reacting to their delivery method.

- Stay calm and focused. Your calmness will help your child regain self-control.
- Teach your child the vocabulary of emotions.
- Never shake a child. Never hit, never spank.
- Put your child in a time-out chair (one minute per year of age).
- Put yourself in a time-out chair.
- Ask yourself: Do I care more about my child's misbehavior right now, or about how she behaves in 10 or 20 years?

Take good care of yourself.

- Be sure to get enough sleep and exercise, and eat healthy.
- Practice tranquility breathing.
- Count to 10 or 100, or backwards from 100 to 10.
- Take some time for yourself each day—a hot bath, soothing music, a walk around the block.

- Get educated about child development and effective parenting.
- Phone a friend. Ask for help, advice, or share a laugh.
- Ask a friend or relative to babysit.
- Give yourself credit for what you are doing right. Remind yourself of what your child is doing right. Write down the things for which you are grateful.
- Remind yourself of the big picture. Difficult times will pass. Your child will change and will eventually grow up.

Handout: Co-Parenting With an Ex-Partner

Sharing children with a former partner can require patience, thoughtfulness, and self-control. Here are recommendations for successful co-parenting:

1. Your child is the priority—not you, not your feelings toward your ex-partner.
2. Focus on *your* relationship with your child—allow your partner to be in charge of *his* relationship with your child.
3. View your relationship with your ex-partner as a business relationship. Be respectful and courteous.
4. Talk to him about your child's specific needs and welfare. Stick to the subject. Don't rehash the problems you've had with each other in the past.
5. Don't bad-mouth your ex-partner, even if he did really bad things. Your child has a right to discover her truth for herself.
6. Don't put your child in the middle. Don't make your child the messenger.
7. Don't make assumptions based on what your child says. Check things out with your ex-partner. Be respectful.
8. When there are disagreements or problems, don't blame. Look for solutions.
9. Respect your ex-partner's privacy. Ignore things that are not your business.
10. Acknowledge your ex-partner for positive things he does. Say thank you.

Coping with parents' divorce can be even more difficult for children than it is for the adults involved. To help your child:

1. Invite conversation. Let her know that her feelings matter. Listen calmly.
2. Help your child put her feelings into words.
3. Legitimize her feelings by how your respond. Listen. Take her seriously. Don't tell her she shouldn't feel that way. Let her know that her feelings are valid, whatever they are.
4. Don't use your child to confide in. Don't ask her to spy on her father for you. Don't ask her to keep secrets from her father. Don't ask questions about her father, his lifestyle, romantic life, money, and so on.
5. Allow your child to love her father. Just like parents have the capacity to love more than one child, children have the capacity to love more than one parent.
6. If she complains about her father, do not join in by also criticizing him. Focus instead on acknowledging *her* feelings.
7. Sometimes children need to ask the same questions over and over. Resist the temptation to get frustrated. This too shall pass.
8. Offer support. Ask: What would help her feel better right now? Drawing? Playing a game? Going on a bike ride?

Section 6 Binder Contents: Inspiration

Suggestions to Therapist

This is included as a separate section in the binder because often women will bring to group poems and inspirational writings they have found and want to share with the other women.

Two handouts provided are

- "Letting Go"
- "Serenity Prayer"

Handout: Letting Go

Letting go means removing our attention from a particular experience or person and putting our focus on the here and now.

Karen Casey

Each Day a New Beginning, reprinted with permission of Hazelden Publishing

"Let Go" Doesn't Mean Stop Caring

To "let go" does not mean stop caring; it means I can't do it for someone else.

To "let go" is not to cut myself off; it's the realization that I can't control another.

To "let go" is not to enable, but to allow learning from natural consequences.

To "let go" is not to try to change or blame another, it is to make the most of myself.

To "let go" is not to care for, but to care about.

To "let go" is not to fix, but to be supportive. It is not to judge, but to allow another to be a human being.

To "let go" is not to be in the middle, arranging all the outcomes, but to allow others to affect their destinies.

To "let go" is not to be protective, it is to permit another to face reality.

To "let go" is not to deny but to accept. It is not to nag, scold or argue with, but instead to search out my own shortcomings and correct them.

To "let go" is not to criticize and regulate anybody, but to try and become what I dream I can be.

To "let go" is not to regret the past, but to grow and live for the future.

To "let go" is to fear less and love more.

Lisa D.

Stepping Stones to Recovery for Young People, reprinted with permission of Hazelden Publishing.

Handout: Serenity Prayer

God, grant me the **serenity**
to accept the things I cannot change ...
the **courage**
to change the things I can ...
and the **wisdom**
to know the difference.

Reinhold Niebuhr

Suggestions to Therapist: Responding to Challenges and Problems

It is virtually impossible to anticipate every possible problem that can arise in doing groups with abusive women. Because they often have significant trauma in their histories, they tend to be resistant to trusting a therapist. While the therapist is in the role of "good momma" to the women, like real life, it is no guarantee that those she cares for will respond.

Even with the best of intentions, a competent therapist may feel overwhelmed or discouraged—especially when women relapse with alcohol, drugs, or violence. At those times, it is important for the therapist to remind herself of the very concepts she teaches in group: she can only be responsible for her own behavior. Through the program, the therapist offers clients an array of options to help them in life. Each woman chooses what she will take with her and what she will leave behind.

My own experience in doing single-gender groups with men and women is that by far, women are much more likely to act out in group, act out against other group members, and generally create more drama. The following list of situations and possible responses is provided to help the therapist think ahead about how she might either deal with them or avoid them altogether.

> **What if** a woman's partner brings her to group and wants to wait in the adjacent waiting room while group is in session, or barges into the room in the middle of group demanding to speak to the woman?
>
> **Answer:** Safety first is the foremost principle in doing these groups—safety for the new client, group members, and therapist. These intrusive boundary violations are the therapist's responsibility to deal with—not the client's. She must stand, go to the partner, and calmly but firmly tell him he must leave the building because it is not appropriate for him to wait next to the group room, and that he may return after group is finished—and wait outside. She then escorts him to the door and locks it after him. When she returns to the group, she must acknowledge that this situation may have been upsetting and ask what reactions the women felt while witnessing it. Women who have been in any type of abusive relationship are likely to experience a resurgence of significant anxiety in response to these situations and must be allowed the opportunity to process their feelings.

What if a woman has a medical emergency during group?

Answer: It is important and helpful to have a landline telephone in a corner of the group room. No matter the nature of the emergency, the therapist must remain in charge and convey calmness. She stops group and addresses the current emergency, tending to the woman in crisis and calling 911 if necessary. When the women in crisis has recovered, left to go home, or been taken by ambulance, what just happened becomes the focus of group discussion. This is what a healthy family does (and what was missing in the family of origin experiences of most of these women): *We talk about what happened and our feelings.*

What if a woman shows up to group smelling of alcohol? Or has difficulty staying awake or appears to be buzzing, under the influence of drugs?

Answer: Sometimes when one person in a room is reeking of alcohol, it may be difficult to ascertain which person it is. In this case, the therapist might simply stop group and say: "I can smell alcohol, like someone has been drinking. I'm wondering if whoever it is that has been drinking would be willing to fess up?" If someone admits to drinking, then the therapist may thank her for her honestly, have her gather her things and leave, and ask her to call the therapist later that day. Coming to group under the influence of alcohol or drugs is a serious violation of the program and is usually an indication that the person has a serious substance abuse problem. The therapist must assess what level of chemical dependency treatment to recommend or require before the woman returns to group. This decision is made in collaboration with the woman's probation officer.

What if she begs the therapist to not tell her probation officer about drinking or drug use?

Answer: The therapist points out that this type of collusion would not be in the woman's overall best interest. She may offer the woman the first chance to come clean with her P.O. before the therapist calls him/her (e.g., 24 hours). The therapist then follows up with the probation officer to make sure that the client was forthright in taking responsibility for her behavior.

What if a woman uses poor judgment in a situation, makes a mistake, and when reporting it to the group, she catastrophizes, characterizing her mistake as drastically worse than it really was (e.g., "This is the end of the world! Here I go again! I've made things so bad, they'll never get better!")? For her, everything is black and white; any setback is a disaster that colors her view of everything else in life.

Answer: Stop her, ask her to describe her feeling cues. Then reframe. Suggest that while she made a mistake, it is a *mistake*—she can learn from it and do things differently next time. The therapist can then refocus her attention on the *lesson* in the mistake. Group members may suggest what the lesson is and often will reveal that they have struggled with similar lessons.

When a woman seems shame-bound, obsessed with berating herself for mistakes, and unable to let go, the therapist might suggest she compartmentalize. This means that instead of thinking about a problem 24/7 or not at all, she budget a set amount of time to think about a problem—and no more (e.g., 20 minutes a day). Twelve-step groups such as Alcoholics Anonymous have wonderful pieces of wisdom for coping with life experiences that can seem overwhelming.

What if a woman is inattentive, interrupts others who are speaking, or makes comments privately to those sitting next to her? What if her cell phone goes off during group?

Answer: These are all inappropriate, disrespectful boundary violations. Sometimes, women who come to group have never been taught appropriate boundaries. Boundaries are essential life skills, and these situations provide teachable moments. Depending on what is happening and how disruptive the woman's behavior is, the therapist might simply say, "Mary, that is inappropriate. Suzy is speaking now and she needs our full, undivided attention and support." Or, at break or the end of the group, the therapist may ask the woman to speak individually with her, note her behavior, and ask what she thinks it conveyed to the rest of the group. Or, in the case of the cell phone, the therapist may tell the woman to gather her things and leave group, especially when a rule has been clearly given that cell phone intrusions are unacceptable and will cause a group member to be dismissed from that group meeting.

What if a woman swears, uses profanity, name calling, racism, men bashing, or sexism?

Answer: These are all disrespectful and inflammatory. As such, they should not be tolerated. When these arise in group, the therapist stops the woman, notes that this language is inappropriate, and asks the woman to rephrase her thoughts. It can also be helpful to ask the group to consider reasons why this language is not appropriate, as part of educating everyone. If the problem persists, the therapist should meet individually with the woman, point out that the problem is continuing and ask her to explain why the therapist has objected in the past. This allows the therapist to be sure that the woman has accurately heard and understands what she has said. If the woman is unwilling to stop, this can be viewed as an indication she is not ready to work on herself (a basic requirement of participation in the program). The therapist then may terminate her from group and refer her back to probation or the court.

What if a woman repeatedly challenges the therapist's authority or continues to disagree or argue with whatever the therapist says? What if she jokes about violence, encourages other women to use violence as a solution to specific problems they share, or asks the therapist what makes her so special that she thinks she can tell everyone what to do? What if the woman tells the therapist that the rest of the group agrees that the therapist is wrong but they are afraid to tell her so?

Answer: How the therapist handles this depends on the context of the challenges. For instance, do the challenges happen during group or outside of group when the woman is speaking individually to the therapist? Initial challenges of the therapist can be therapeutic opportunities, but ongoing challenges usually indicate that a woman is not appropriate to the program. It is the therapist's responsibility to maintain the integrity of the program and the group. Ongoing challenges by a woman who is not ready to work on herself can be poisonous to the group. In those cases, the woman may be offered the option of working individually with the therapist (in lieu of group) or terminated from the program and referred back to probation or the court.

What if a group member threatens or intimidates another group member? What if a group member threatens the therapist?

Answer: On the one hand, this can be extremely distressing and destructive to the group. On the other hand, this can provide valuable opportunities to learn—for the group members as well as the therapist. How a therapist chooses to respond depends on many factors (e.g., context, motivation of hostile person, apparent impact on other person and group, whether this is the first time or a subsequent one, whether it has been addressed before in group, whether the woman appears to be under the influence of chemicals, how far into the group meeting the confrontation happens).

In all cases, the safety of the group is of primary importance. Sometimes, the safest choice may be for the therapist to help the angry woman to restate and process her feelings and the reason for her hostility. Then help the victim find her voice and respectfully respond. Last, have the group process feelings about what just happened. Always, the therapist must set limits on group members' behavior and insist that threats and intimidation are violent and inappropriate. The therapist must maintain the safety of the group. On some occasions, the safest and most responsible action is to dismiss the threatening woman from group.

As with what happens in a healthy family, hostility and anger are acknowledged and addressed; each member has a right to express her own opinion and feelings; even when those are different than others, each member has a right to be treated with respect. The therapist's willingness to be authentic and humble will go far in gaining the respect of the women as well as modeling important qualities.

What if if a woman decompensates, dissociates, or experiences flashbacks in group?

Answer: If this happens, everyone else in the group will also be keenly aware of this. The most therapeutic response is to gently stop the group and tend to the woman who is having trouble. In a gentle, quiet voice, the therapist may kneel in front of the woman, moving into her field of vision. Acknowledge that she appears to be having a hard time. Ask if something is going on right now that is upsetting her? Ask if she can hear her voice. Reassure her that she is safe and not in danger, that she is here, in this room, with the therapist, with the group. "Let's try to bring you back to the room, OK? Where are we, what time is it? Can you describe the room?" Ask her to focus attention on the feeling of the chair underneath her or her feet on the floor. "Come back into the room and be present. Hear the quietness of the room. You are safe here. You are with friends."

Sometimes the woman will be able to later speak about what she was experiencing and other times she may not want to. Either way, it is important to spend time individually with the woman after group to evaluate her safety in leaving. What will she do after group? Will she go home? Can she drive? How can she take care of herself? Does she have a support system? It is also recommended that the therapist call the woman later in the day to check on her.

What if a group member is always interrupting others, talking over them?

Answer: While it can be good to have group members who are eager to participate in discussion, more shy women may feel slighted or use this as an excuse to avoid participating. It is important that all group members view the group as a supportive, helpful resource.

The first time this happens, the therapist may firmly remind the woman of the rules about not interrupting, that she must raise her hand, wait to be called on, take turns. If it happens again, the therapist may speak individually to the woman at break or after group. She may acknowledge that the woman wants to participate—a good thing—but that interrupting is rude and cannot continue. The therapist may then make more effort to reach out to quieter group members, directly asking them for thoughts on the topic that is being addressed.

What if a woman responds minimally, does not participate in discussions, or looks bored and inattentive?

Answer: The therapist may speak to her individually at break or after group, asking how she is feeling being in group and pointing out that she rarely speaks in group and often looks bored. Sometimes women feel anxious about group or preoccupied about life outside of group. Finding out the reason behind the behavior can help the therapist better know how to encourage her to participate.

What if a woman says she doesn't think she should have to do the journal homework because she never gets angry anymore?

Answer: Homework is *mandatory, not optional.* The therapist may refer her to the binder handout that explains how to do the homework. Or, the therapist may ask other group members to offer suggestions about situations to process in the homework exercise. This can be a good time to remind group members that the purpose of the program is *not* to eliminate their anger (a healthy and important emotion), but rather to help them be more self-aware and capable of making wise choices in how they behave when they are angry. It can also be helpful to periodically ask every group member to share an entry from her journal homework, processing it with the group.

What if the therapist is feeling really frustrated and inadequate, that nothing she is trying to accomplish in group is working or helpful?

Answer: This can be a common experience of even the most seasoned clinicians. Questions she can ask herself include the following: Am I working harder than my clients? Am I expecting unrealistic results? Am I addressing my goals, or my clients' goals? Have I lost sight of what my clients want from therapy? Am I assuming too much responsibility for my clients? Am I not expecting enough?

This is a helpful cue for the therapist to discuss these questions with respected colleagues. It can also be a valuable intervention to share these questions with the group and ask for their feedback about the group experience. This type of discussion can help a group coalesce as a community and facilitate members' deeper self-reflection.

Appendix A: Additional Resources

Books for Clinicians

The following books are recommended for therapists who want to deepen their understanding of the many issues related to domestic violence. They are listed in addition to the chapter references in Appendix B.

Women's Violence and Domestic Violence

Anderson, P., & Struckman-Johnson, C. (1998). *Sexually aggressive women: Current perspectives and controversies.* New York: Guilford Press.

Cook, P. (1997). *Abused men: The hidden side of domestic violence.* Westport, CT: Praeger.

Dutton, D. (2006). *Rethinking domestic violence.* Vancouver: UBC Press.

Gelles, R. J., & Straus, M. A. (1988). *Intimate violence: The causes and consequences of abuse in the American family.* New York: Touchstone.

Hamel, J. (2005). *Gender inclusive treatment of intimate partner abuse: A comprehensive approach.* New York: Springer.

Hamel, J., & Nicholls, T. (2007). *Family interventions in domestic violence: A handbook of gender-inclusive theory and treatment.* New York: Springer.

Miller, S. (2005). *Victims as offenders: The paradox of women's violence in relationships.* New Brunswick, NJ: Rutgers University Press.

Mills, L. (2003). *Insult to injury: Rethinking our responses to intimate abuse.* Princeton, NJ: Princeton University Press.

Pearson, P. (1997). *When she was bad: Violent women and the myth of innocence.* New York: Viking.

Pence, E., & Paymar, M. (1993). *Education groups for men who batter: The Duluth model.* New York: Springer Publishing.

Straus, M. A., & Gelles, R. (1990). *Physical violence in American families.* New Brunswick, NJ: Transaction Publishers.

Straus, M., Gelles, R., & Steinmetz, S. (2006). *Behind closed doors: Violence in the American family.* 2nd ed. New Brunswick, NJ: Transaction Publishers.

Walker, L. (1984). *The battered woman syndrome.* New York: Springer.

Attachment Theory and Treatment

Cassidy, J., & Shaver, P.R. (Eds.). (1999). *Handbook of attachment: Theory, research, and clinical applications*. New York: Guilford Press.

Flores, P. (2004). *Addiction as an attachment disorder*. Lanhan, MD: Jason Aronson.

Karen, R. (1998). *Becoming attached: First relationships and how they shape our capacity to love*. New York: Oxford University Press.

Stosny, S. (1995). *Treating attachment abuse: A compassionate approach*. New York: Springer.

Motivational Interviewing

Miller, W., & Rollnick, S. (2002). *Motivational interviewing: Preparing people for change*. New York: Guilford Press.

Personality Disorders and Treatment

American Psychiatric Association. (2000). *Diagnostic and statistical manual of the American Psychiatric Association IV-TR*. Washington, DC: Author.

Magnavita, J. (1997). *Restructuring personality disorders: A short-term dynamic approach*. New York: Guilford Press.

Trauma Theory and Treatment

Briere, J., & Scott, C. (2006). *Principles of trauma therapy: A guide to symptoms, evaluation and treatment*. Thousand Oaks, CA: Sage Publications.

Herman, J. L. (1992). *Trauma and recovery: The aftermath of violence—From domestic abuse to political terror*. New York: Basic Books.

Relationships

Gottman, J. (1994). *Why marriages succeed or fail ... and how you can make yours last*. New York: Fireside.

Gottman, J., & Silver, N. (1999). *The seven principles for making marriage work*. New York: Three Rivers Press.

Books for Clients

Before recommending any book or resource to a client, the therapist should already have read the book or reviewed the Website to ensure that the information is appropriate to the client's needs.

DeAngelis, B. (1994.) *Are you the one for me? Knowing who's right and avoiding who's wrong.* New York: Dell Publishing.

Evans, P. (1992). *The verbally abusive relationship: How to recognize it and how to respond.* Holbrook, MA: Adams Media Corp.

Gottman, J. (1994). *Why marriages succeed or fail … and how you can make yours last.* New York: Fireside.

Gottman, J., & Silver, N. (1999). *The seven principles for making marriage work.* New York: Three Rivers Press.

Katherine, A. (1991). *Boundaries: Where you end and I begin. How to recognize and set healthy boundaries.* Park Ridge, IL: Parkside Publishing Corp.

Moskovitz, R. (1996). *Lost in the mirror: An inside look at borderline personality disorder.* Dallas, TX: Taylor Publishing Co.

Ruiz, D. M. (2001). *The four agreements: A practical guide to personal freedom (A Toltec wisdom book).* San Rafael, CA: Amber-Allen Publishing.

Smedes, L. B. (1984). *Forgive and forget: Healing the hurts we don't deserve.* New York: Pocket Books (Simon and Schuster).

Smedes, L. B. (1996). *The art of forgiving: When you need to forgive and don't know how.* New York: Ballantine Books (Random House).

Websites

California Department of Alcohol and Drug Programs: www.adp.ca.gov
See this Website for *Methamphetamine Treatment: A Practitioner's Reference 2007.* This document provides important information about methamphetamine assessment, treatment, and recovery with additional information about use among women.

Domestic Abuse Helpline for Men and Women: DAHMW.org or (888)7HELPLINE (888-743-5754).
Provides a 24-hour hotline operated by staff and trained volunteers to offer information and crisis intervention to victims of intimate partner abuse.

The Forgiveness Project: www.theforgivenessproject.com
A Website that offers a forum for examining the complexities, difficulties, and value of forgiveness.

Hazelden: www.Hazelden.org
    In addition to providing residential treatment for substance abuse,
    Hazelden provides an extensive catalog of educational materials for liv-
    ing a clean and sober life.
Los Angeles Gay Center: lagaycenter.org
    Provides information, referral, education, and counseling services for
    LGBT domestic violence survivors and abusers, and advocacy, consulta-
    tion, and training for law enforcement, criminal justice personnel, ser-
    vice providers, and so forth.
National Council on Alcoholism and Drug Dependence: www.NCADD.
    org or (800)622-2255
    Provides contact information for local treatment resources and educa-
    tional materials on alcoholism and drug dependence.
National Institute on Alcohol Abuse and Alcoholism: www.NIAAA.nih.
    gov or (301)443-3860
    Information and publications on all aspects of alcohol abuse and alcohol-
    ism, including *The Motivational Enhancement Therapy Manual* (part of the
    Project Match Series). Many publications are also available in Spanish.
Prevent Child Abuse America: www.preventchildabuse.org or (312)663-3520
    This organization provides an array of easy-to-understand educational
    materials on topics such as positive parenting, child abuse awareness,
    discipline, child development, sexual abuse, and stress management.
    Many publications are available to download or purchase directly. Many
    are also available in Spanish.
Stop Abuse for Everyone: http://www.SAFE4all.org or (503)853-8686
    An organization that provides services, publications, and training to
    people who often fall between the cracks of domestic violence services:
    straight men, gays, lesbians, teens, and the elderly.

Movies/Media

20/20: Battered Husbands
    Episode aired February 7, 2003. Can be ordered from ABCNEWS@data-
    pakservices.com or by calling (800)505-6139. Examines societal messages
    minimizing women's violence. Interviews men who have been abused
    and a woman in recovery from her violence in previous relationships.
Men Don't Tell
    CBS made-for-TV movie (1993) starring Peter Strauss and Judith Light
    tells the fictionalized account of an abused man. The movie rights are
    owned by Lorimar Productions, which has not yet made the movie avail-
    able for video purchase. However, occasionally it may be rebroadcast on
    a cable channel.

Windows of Opportunity
Thirteen-minute video produced and distributed through the California Attorney General's Office, through the Safe from the Start Program. This and other education materials about the impact of domestic violence on children are available for order at www.safefromthestart.org. Orders placed from outside California may require a nominal fee.

Support Groups

AlAnon Family Group Headquarters: www.alanon.alateen.org or (888) 4AL-ANON (425-2666)
  Provides information and makes referrals to local support groups for partners and other significant adults in an alcoholic person's life. Alateen groups offer support to children of alcoholics.
Alcoholics Anonymous (AA) World Services: www.aa.org or (212)870-3400
  Makes referrals to local AA groups and provides informational materials on the AA 12-step program.
Narcotics Anonymous (NA): www.na.org or (818)773-9999
  Information and referral to local support groups for persons with drug abuse or dependence. Follows 12-step program similar to AA's.
National Association for Children of Alcoholics (NACoA): www.ncoa.net or (888)554-COAS
  Works on behalf of children of alcoholic or drug-dependent parents.
Overeaters Anonymous (OA): www.oa.org or (505)891-2664
  Information and referral to local support groups for persons struggling with compulsive overeating or other eating disorders. Follows 12-step program similar to AA's.
Sex and Love Addicts Anonymous: http://72.52.143.94/ or (210)828-7900
  Information and referral to local support groups for persons who want help with destructive consequences related to sex addiction, love addiction, and so forth. Follows 12-step program similar to AA's.

Local Resources That May Be Available in Your Community

Legal aid services
District attorney
Law enforcement (police and sheriff's department may provide advocates to support victims through court process)
Family court—Mediation, family law facilitator, family law advocate

Appendix B: References

Chapter 1

Abel, E. M. (1999, July). *Who are women in batterer intervention programs: Implications for practice*. Paper presented at the 6th International Family Violence Research Conference, Durham, NH.

Archer, J. (2000). Sex differences in aggression between heterosexual partners: A meta-analytic review. *Psychological Bulletin, 126*, 651–680.

Archer, J. (2002). Sex differences in physically aggressive acts between heterosexual partners: A meta-analytic review. *Aggression and Violent Behavior, 7*, 313–351.

Bachman, R., & Carmody, D. C. (1994). Fighting fire with fire: The effects of victim resistance in intimate versus stranger perpetrated assaults against females. *Journal of Family Violence, 9*, 317–331.

Carney, M. M., Buttell, F., & Dutton, D. (2007). Women who perpetrate intimate partner violence: A review of the literature with recommendations for treatment. *Aggression and Violent Behavior, 12*, 108–115.

Dutton, D., Nicholls, T., & Spidel, A. (2005). Female perpetrators of intimate abuse. In F. Buttell & M. M. Carney (Eds.), *Women who perpetrate relationship violence: Moving beyond political correctness* (pp. 1–31). New York: Haworth Press.

Feld, S. L., & Straus, M. A. (1989). Escalation and desistance of wife assault in marriage. *Criminology 17*, 141–161.

Ferraro, K., & Moe, A. (2003). Mothering, crime and incarceration. *Journal of Ethnography, 32*, 9–23.

Fiebert, M. S., & Gonzalez, D. M. (1997). Women who initiate assaults: The reasons offered for such behavior. *Psychological Reports, 80*, 583–590.

Gelles, R. J., & Straus, M. A. (1988). *Intimate violence: The causes and consequences of abuse in the American family*. New York: Touchstone.

Henning, K., Jones, A., & Holford, R. (2003). Treatment needs of women arrested for domestic violence: A comparison with male offenders. *Journal of Interpersonal Violence, 18*, 839–856.

Hines, D. A., Brown, J., & Dunning, E. (2003). *Characteristics of callers to the domestic abuse helpline for men*. Durham, NH: University of New Hampshire, Family Violence Lab.

Holtzworth-Munroe, A. (2005). Female perpetration of physical aggression against an intimate partner: A controversial new topic of study. *Violence and Victims, 20*, 251–259.

Laroche, D. (2005). *Aspects of the context and consequences of domestic violence— Situational couple violence and intimate terrorism in Canada in 1999.* Quebec City: Government of Quebec. Translated by James Lawler.

Mullings, J., Hartley, D., & Marquet, J. (2004). Exploring the relationship between alcohol use, childhood maltreatment, and treatment needs among female prisoners. *Substance Use and Misuse, 39,* 277–305.

Rennison, C., & Welchans, S. (2000). *Intimate partner violence.* Bureau of Justice Statistics Report (NCJ 178247). Washington, DC: U.S. Department of Justice.

Straus, M. A. (1997). Physical assaults by women partners: A major social problem. In M. R. Walsh (Ed.), *Women, men and gender: Ongoing debates* (pp. 210–221). New Haven, CT: Yale University Press.

Straus, M. A. (1999). *Controversy over domestic violence by women: A methodological, theoretical, and sociology of science analysis.* National Institute of Mental Health Report (NCJ 16243). Washington, DC: U.S. Department of Health and Human Services.

Straus, M. A., & Gelles, R. (1990). *Physical violence in American families.* New Brunswick, NJ: Transaction Publishers.

Straus, M. A., Gelles, R., & Steinmetz, S. (1980). *Behind closed doors: Violence in the American family.* Newbury Park, CA: Sage.

Tannen, D. (1990). *You just don't understand.* New York: Ballentine.

Chapter 2

Ainsworth, M.D., Blehar M. C., Waters, F., & Wall, S. (1978). *Patterns of attachment: A psychological study of the strange situation.* Hillsdale, NJ: Erlbaum.

Bookwala, J. (2002). The role of own and perceived partner attachment in relationship aggression. *Journal of Interpersonal Violence, 17,* 84–100.

Bowlby, J. (1969). *Attachment: Vol. 1. Attachment and loss* (2nd ed.). London: Hogarth Press.

Bowlby, J. (1973). *Separation: Anxiety and anger* Vol. 2. New York: Basic Books.

Bowlby, J. (1980). *Loss, Sadness, and depression:* Vol. 3. *Attachment and loss.* New York: Basic Books.

Briere, J., & Scott, C. (2006). *Principles of trauma therapy: A guide to symptoms, evaluation and treatment.* Thousand Oaks, CA: Sage Publications.

Hazen, C., & Shaver, P. (1987). Conceptualizing romantic love as an attachment process. *Journal of Personality and Social Psychology, 52,* 511–524.

Main, M. (1999). Attachment theory: Eighteen points with suggestions for future studies. In J. Cassidy & P. R. Shaver (Eds.), *Handbook of attachment: Theory, research, and clinical applications* (pp. 355–377). New York: Guilford Press.

Perry, B. (1997). Incubated in terror: Neurodevelopmental factors in the "cycle of violence." In J. D. Osofsky (Ed.), *Children in a violent society* pp. 124–148. New York: Guilford Press.

Walker, L. (1984). *The battered woman syndrome.* New York: Springer.

Chapter 3

Prochaska, J., DiClemente, C., & Norcross, C. (1992). In search of how people change: Applications to addictive behaviors. *American Psychologist, 47,* 1102–1127.

Chapter 4

American Psychiatric Association. (2000). *Diagnostic and statistical manual of mental disorders* (4 ed., text rev.). Washington, DC: Author.

California Department of Alcohol and Drug Programs. (2007). *Methamphetamine treatment: A practitioner's reference 2007.*

Ewing, J. A. (1984). Detecting alcoholism: The CAGE questionnaire. *JAMA, 252,* 1905–1907.

Chapter 10

Goleman, D. (2006, October). Interview: Meeting of the minds. *"O" Magazine,* pp. 251–256.

Gottmen, J, (1994). Why marriages succeed or fail … and how you can make yours last. New York: Fireside.

Stosny, S. (1995). *Treating attachment abuse: A compassionate approach.* New York: Springer.

Walker, L. (1984). *The battered woman syndrome.* New York: Springer.

Index

.

Printed in the United States
by Baker & Taylor Publisher Services